The New Hypnodontics

Advances And Applications Of Clinical
Hypnosis In Modern Dentistry

© 2024 Cristóbal Schilling, Catalina Bascuñan First Edition

ISBN:

CHC Editions

Nueva Providencia 2211 Of.818, Providencia

Santiago - Chile.

Contact us:

Mail: contacto@hipnosisclinica.cl Web: www.hipnosisclinica.cl

Printed in Chile/Printed in Chile

All rights reserved.

This publication may not be reproduced in whole or in part, or recorded in, or transmitted by any information retrieval system, in any form or by any means, mechanical, photochemical, electronic, magnetic, electro-optical, photocopying or otherwise without prior written permission from the Publisher.

PS. CRISTÓBAL SCHILLING

CATALINA BASCUÑAN

The New Hypnodontics

Advances And Applications Of Clinical Hypnosis In Modern Dentistry

EDITORIAL

CLINICAL HYPNOSIS CENTER

INDEX

INDEX	7
INTRODUCTION	11
BACKGROUND OF HYPNOSIS	11
HYPNOSIS IN THE MODERN ERA	14
HYPNOSIS IN DENTISTRY	15
CHAPTER 2: BASICS OF HYPNOSIS	25
WHAT IS HYPNOSIS?	25
HOW HYPNOSIS WORKS	28
PRINCIPLES OF HYPNOSIS	34
SUGGESTION AS A PRINCIPLE OF HYPNOSIS	37
RELAXATION AS A PRINCIPLE OF HYPNOSIS	48
RAPPORT	61
THE EXPECTATION	67
IMAGINATION AS THE PRINCIPLE OF HYPNOSIS	75
MYTHS AND FACTS ABOUT HYPNOSIS	82
STYLES OF HYPNOSIS	83
HYPNOSIS TECHNIQUES	87
THE SCIENCE BEHIND INDUCTION	
OF GAZE FIXATION	91

DEEPENING TECHNIQUES	94
SUGGESTION TECHNIQUES	101
WHO CAN BE HYPNOTIZED?	106
EFFICACY AND SAFETY OF HYPNOSIS	107
HYPNOTIC ANCHORAGE	108
CHAPTER 3: THE PROCESS OF HYPNOSIS IN DENTISTRY	**113**
PATIENT EVALUATION	113
CHAPTER 4: APPLICATIONS OF HYPNOSIS IN DENTISTRY	**121**
RELAXATION AND STRESS MANAGEMENT	121
HYPNOTIC ANALGESIA	137
ANXIETY MANAGEMENT	148
DENTAL PHOBIA	151
EMETIC REFLEX CONTROL	157
BRUXISM	163
DECREASE IN BLEEDING	175
DISCOMFORT DURING DENTAL CLEANING	182
REDUCTION OF EXCESSIVE SALIVATION	187
ADAPTATION TO DENTAL APPLIANCES SUCH AS PROSTHESES, ORTHODONTICS, RETAINERS AND OTHER	192
PEDIATRIC DENTAL HYPNOSIS	199
SPECIFIC BENEFITS OF HYPNOSIS IN CHILDREN	217
A. STORYTELLING	217
B. GUIDED IMAGINATION	221
C. POSITIVE SUGGESTIONS	226
D. RELAXATION TRAINING	231
E. POST-HYPNOTIC SUGGESTIONS	234
ANXIETY AND FEAR REDUCTION	237
RELAXATION TECHNIQUES	238
RELAXATION VISUALIZATION	240
1. DISPLAY	240
POSITIVE SUGGESTIONS	248
STORYTELLING	253

THE NEW HYPNODONTICS	9
RELIEF OF PAIN AND DISCOMFORT	261
PROMOTION OF HEALTHY ORAL HYGIENE HABITS	269
STEPS OF A HYPNOSIS TO PROMOTE DENTAL HYGIENE	271
MANAGEMENT OF SPECIFIC PROBLEMS	272
ETHICS IN HYPNODONTICS	280
APPENDIX	291
1 - ANNEX ADULTS	291
2. ANNEX CHILDREN	304
BIBLIOGRAPHY	325

INTRODUCTION

The application of hypnosis in the field of dentistry, or hypnodontics, has become increasingly popular in modern dental practice. In this introduction, we will explore the historical background of hypnosis, its development and application in the field of medicine and, in particular, in dentistry.

BACKGROUND OF THE HYPNOSIS

Origins of Hypnosis

Hypnosis, as we know it today, is a technique that focuses on inducing an altered state of consciousness to facilitate therapeutic change. However, the origins of hypnosis go back to ancient civilizations, long before psychology or formal medicine identified and developed it as a discipline in its own right.

The earliest indications of practices resembling hypnosis can be found in the ritual and healing traditions of primitive cultures. The shamans and spiritual leaders of these societies, such as the ancient Egyptians, Greeks, and Persians, often used hypnosis during their healing ceremonies and rituals. These rituals often involved the induction of altered states of consciousness through techniques such as chanting, dancing, rhythm and meditation. Although these practices were not recognized as hypnosis at the time, they laid the early foundations for what would become the method used in the modern era (Krippner, 2002; Gauld, 1992).

In the 18th century, interest in these altered states of consciousness began to take shape in the academic and scientific world. Franz Anton Mesmer, an Austrian physician, is often considered one of the forerunners of hypnosis, although his theory of "animal magnetism" and his methods of "magnetic healing" were considered pseudo-science in his time. However, Mesmer was one of the first to use relaxation and suggestion techniques to induce altered states of consciousness, thus laying the groundwork for what would later become known as hypnosis (Crabtree, 1993).

As we moved into the 19th century, physicians and scientists began to develop a deeper and more formalized understanding of hypnosis. James Braid, a Scottish physician, was the first to use the term "hypno- sis," derived from the Greek god of sleep, Hypnos. Braid saw hypnosis as a state of purposeful focus and concentration, quite distinct from ordinary sleep. His work was crucial in establishing hypnosis as a serious and valid technique in the field of medicine and psychology (Yeates, 2018).

Hypnosis has continued to evolve and refine since then, benefiting from the growing scientific understanding of human psychology and the mind. Although its use in dentistry is a relatively recent phenomenon, hypnodontics builds on this long history of development and adaptation. The hypnotic techniques used in dental care today are based on these centuries of research and practice, demonstrating once again that hypnosis, as a technique and therapeutic tool, has deep roots in human history (Heap & Aravind, 2002).

In summary, hypnosis is a therapeutic technique that has evolved over the centuries and is based on ancient practices of trance and suggestion. Since its appearance in modern medicine, hypnosis has been the subject of study and has been recognized as a serious and valid technique in the treatment of various conditions. The sources mentioned above provide reliable and rigorous information about the history of hypnosis and its evolution over time.

HYPNOSIS IN THE MODERN ERA

During the twentieth century, hypnosis began to gain greater acceptance and legitimacy in the medical and psychological world. Researchers and mental health practitioners, such as Milton Erickson and Dave Elman, contributed greatly to this advance. Elman, in particular, popularized rapid induction techniques, and Erickson developed nontraditional, often indirect, approaches that became the basis for what is now known as Ericksonian hypnosis (Heap & Aravind, 2002).

Clinical psychology and medicine began to exploit and document its benefits for a variety of conditions, from pain management to the treatment of sleep disorders and anxiety. Scientific studies began to provide an empirical basis for the efficacy of hypnosis, and neuroscientific research findings began to unravel the underlying mechanisms that make hypnosis work at the brain level (Smith, 2011).

Today, it remains a widely used and accepted therapeutic technique in medicine and clinical psychology. Hypnotic techniques have been adapted and modified to accommodate a variety of therapeutic needs, and hypnosis continues to be the subject of scientific research and debate in the medical and scientific community (Heap & Aravind, 2002).

In summary, hypnosis has undergone a significant advance in the 20th century, thanks to the contribution of researchers and mental health professionals. It has been the object of study and has been recognized as a serious and valid technique in the treatment of various conditions. The sources mentioned above provide reliable and rigorous information about the evolution of hypnosis in the 20th century and its use in medicine and clinical psychology.

HYPNOSIS AT ODONTOLOGY

History and Development of Hypnodontics

While hypnosis itself has been practiced and studied for centuries, its application in dentistry is a relatively recent phenomenon. Hypnodontics, as it is known today, has its roots in the last decades of the 20th century and has continued to evolve throughout the 21st century.

Its rise in the field of dentistry can be attributed, in part, to advances in the understanding of the human mind and the development of more sophisticated hypnosis techniques. However, there have also been key figures in dentistry who have played an important role in the promotion and development of hypnodontics.

Among them, Dr. Aaron Moss (1997) is particularly noteworthy. In the 1980s, Dr. Moss began exploring hypnosis as a tool for managing patient anxiety and fear in the dental clinic. With an extensive background in psychology, Dr. Moss was one of the first dentists to effectively integrate hypnosis into dental practice. His efforts helped legitimize hypnosis in the field of dentistry and paved the way for its wider adoption.

Hypnosis is currently used in dentistry to help patients manage anxiety and fear of dental procedures, control pain and discomfort, reduce the gag reflex, and improve postoperative recovery, among other applications. Hypnosis techniques can also be used to promote positive oral hygiene behaviors and to facilitate treatment in patients with dental phobias or with difficulties cooperating with dental procedures.

Although hypnosis in dentistry is still in its early stages compared with other applications of hypnosis, research and clinical practice are beginning to demonstrate its potential. Studies indicate that hypnosis can be a useful adjunct to conventional dental treatments, and hypnosis training is becoming increasingly popular among dentists and other dental health professionals.

The field of hypnodontics continues to evolve, with new research deepening our understanding of how hypnosis works and how it can be applied more effectively in dentistry. As more and more practitioners embrace hypnosis and integrate it into their practice, it is becoming increasingly clear that hypnosis has an important role to play in the future of dental treatment.

This book sets out to explore in detail how hypnosis is used in dentistry, the specific techniques and approaches employed, and how it can benefit both dentists and patients. Through a comprehensive review of the history, theory, and practice of hypnodontics, we hope to shed light on this fascinating and promising area of dentistry.

The Legacy of Aaron Moss in Hypnodontics

Aaron Moss, M.D., is a notable name in the evolution of hypnodontics. A dentist by profession, but also trained in psychology, Moss was one of the first practitioners to recognize and capitalize on the potential of hypnosis in these treatments.

Dental anxiety is a common and significant problem. It is estimated that a considerable proportion of the population suffers from some degree of dental anxiety, which can range from mild discomfort to extreme fear of receiving dental treatment. This can lead patients to avoid visiting the dentist, which in turn can result in poor oral health and an increased risk of serious dental problems.

Dr. Aaron Moss, aware of this problem, sought alternative solutions to combat dental anxiety, and his exploration led him to hypnosis. Moss recognized that hypnosis, with its ability to influence emotional states and perception, had great potential to trans- form the dental experience of anxious patients.

Moss developed a number of hypnotic induction techniques that were specifically suited to the dental setting. These included methods to help patients enter a state of hypnosis quickly and effectively, which was essential given the limited time for dental appointments. The induction methods used by Moss a menu- do included visualization, concentration and progressive body relaxation, allowing patients to reach a state of calm and serenity.

Beyond induction techniques, Moss also developed a series of hypnotic suggestions aimed at reducing anxiety and fear in patients. These often focused on changing patients' perceptions of dental procedures, encouraging more positive thoughts and emotions rather than fear and apprehension.

For example, it could suggest that patients would experience dental procedures as comfortable and relaxing, or that they would feel a sense of detachment or disconnection from the procedure itself. These suggestions, re- forced by hypnosis, could change the way patients experienced and responded to dental procedures.

Moss hypnosis techniques have shown significant efficacy in managing dental anxiety and improving the patient's experience in the dental clinic. Furthermore, these techniques can also reduce the need for anesthesia and pain medication, which can improve patient safety and well-being.

In summary, hypnosis has proven to be a valuable tool for the management of dental anxiety, and the techniques developed by Dr. Aaron Moss have been especially effective. These techniques can help patients overcome their fear and anxiety, which can significantly improve their oral health and quality of life.

Moss's work showed that patients who received hypnosis before and during dental procedures reported significantly lower levels of anxiety compared to those who did not receive hypnosis. This not only made the dental treatment experience more pleasant for patients, but also may have contributed to better oral health outcomes by making patients more willing to seek and receive dental treatment.

Moss's work in managing dental anxiety with hypnosis has had a lasting impact on the field of dentistry, and his techniques and approaches continue to be used and developed by dentists to this day. His legacy serves as a powerful reminder of how the tools and techniques of psychology can be used to improve dental care and patient health.

Pain management is one of the most critical challenges in any branch of medicine, and dentistry is no exception. Often, the fear of experiencing pain during dental procedures is what drives dental anxiety. Dr. Aaron Moss, aware of this connection intrinsic, he set his sights on the management of dental pain through hypnosis. His goal was not only to alleviate patients' suffering, but also to minimize the use of pharmacological anesthesia, which can sometimes have undesirable side effects.

In this way he developed hypnotic suggestion techniques specifically designed to induce analgesia (reduction of pain) and anesthesia (absence of sensation). Some of these suggestions involved patients visualizing their mouth and teeth as anesthetized or insensitive to pain. Other suggestions focused on dissociation, encouraging patients to imagine that they were in a nice, quiet place away from the dental office.

These techniques varied in their approach, but all had the same goal: to change the patient's perception of pain. In doing so, these suggestions could have an analgesic and anesthetic effect, allowing them to endure dental procedures with minimal or no discomfort.

The results of the Moss techniques were remarkable. Patients who underwent hypnosis reported a significant decrease in pain and discomfort during and after dental procedures. This decrease was so pronounced that Moss was able to perform dental procedures with minimal or no pharmacologic anesthesia.

This had a double benefit. First, it improved the patient experience, as they not only experienced less pain, but also avoided the potential side effects of pharmacologic anesthesia. Second, it allowed Moss to perform procedures more quickly and with fewer interruptions, as he did not have to administer anesthesia and wait for it to take effect.

Moss's approach to dental pain control has had a lasting impact on dentistry. His techniques have been adopted and adapted by many dentists and have helped establish hypnosis as a viable and effective tool for pain management in dentistry. Thus, Moss's legacy lives on in modern dental practices and continues to benefit patients around the world.

Moss's impact on the field of hypnodontics was not limited to his own patients or his own practice. Recognizing the importance of hypnosis training for dental professionals, he extended his influence beyond his practice through the education and training of other dentists.

He was a fervent advocate of continuing education in dentistry. In particular, he strongly believed in the need for dentists to be trained in hypnosis techniques to improve patient care. As such, he devoted a significant part of his career to the training of other dental professionals.

Through a series of workshops and seminars, he provided training in hypnodontics to dentists from around the world. These training events covered a wide range of topics, from basic hypnotic induction techniques to more advanced applications of hypnosis in the management of dental pain and anxiety.

Moss' workshops and seminars were known for their hands-on approach. In addition, he believed in the importance of experiential learning and therefore ensured that his workshops included ample opportunities for practice and experimentation.

Moss' efforts in hypnodontic training,

had a lasting impact. He trained a generation of dentists in the techniques of hypnosis, many of whom continue to use these techniques in their practice today. Through his teaching, he extended the reach of hypnosis, allowing more patients to benefit from this valuable therapeutic tool.

In summary, Moss' contributions to hypnodontics have been invaluable. Through his clinical practice, he demonstrated the efficacy of hypnosis in the management of anxiety and dental pain. Through his teaching, he trained a generation of dentists in the use of hypnosis, ensuring that his techniques and approaches continue to benefit patients long after his own career. His commitment to training and education has helped legitimize hypnosis in the field of dentistry and has left a lasting legacy that remains relevant today.

Medical Advances and Applications

As hypnosis gained acceptance in the twentieth century, its application expanded beyond the confines of mere suggestion and entertainment. The disciplines of psychology and medicine began to explore the therapeutic potential of hypnosis, leading to numerous applications that have fundamentally changed the way we treat a variety of health conditions.

One of the earliest medical uses of hypnosis was in the treatment of pain. During World War I and World War II, physicians used hypnosis to treat soldiers with traumatic pain on the battlefield when conventional anesthetics were unavailable or insufficient. The promising results of these early applications laid the groundwork for the development of hypnoanesthesia and hypnoanalgesia, techniques that have been used since then.

use hypnosis to induce anesthesia and relieve pain without the use of drugs.

Hypnosis has also found its place in the field of psychotherapy. Psychiatrist Milton Erickson was a pioneer in the use of hypnosis in therapy, and his flexible and indirect approach changed the way it is practiced. Ericksonian hypnosis, as it is now known, uses suggestion and metaphor to help individuals tap into their unconscious and discover new ways of thinking and behaving. Today, hypnosis is used in psychotherapy to treat a variety of conditions, from anxiety disorders and depression to addictions and eating disorders.

Beyond pain management and psychotherapy, hypnosis has been used in a number of other medical applications. These include management of irritable bowel syndrome, treatment of migraine headaches, management of nausea and vomiting associated with chemotherapy, improvement of recovery after surgery, and facilitation of childbirth.

Advances in neuroscience have played a crucial role in the consolidation of hypnosis in modern medicine. Neuroimaging techniques, such as functional magnetic resonance imaging (fMRI) and electroencephalography (EEG), have allowed researchers to explore what happens in the brain during this treatment. These studies have shown that hypnosis can alter brain activity in specific and predictable ways, providing a scientific basis for its efficacy.

For example, research has shown that it can increase activity in the areas of the brain associated with attention and concentration, and decrease activity in the areas of the brain associated with attention and concentration, and decrease activity in the areas of the brain associated with attention and concentration, and decrease activity in the areas of the brain associated with attention and concentration.

areas associated with self-awareness and critical evaluation. This change in brain activity can facilitate suggestion and enable deeper changes in individuals' thoughts, emotions, and behaviors (El- kins, G. R. 2015).

Despite these advances, hypnosis still has great unexplored potential. As we continue to deepen our understanding of the human mind and brain, we are likely to discover new ways to use it to improve health and well-being. Dentistry, as we will see throughout this book, is one of the many areas in which hypnosis is beginning to make a significant di- ference.

Hypnosis in the 21st Century: New Frontiers

The 21st century has seen an explosion of interest and research in hypnosis. With the advancement of technology and neuroimaging techniques, we now have unprecedented insight into how hypnosis affects the brain and how we can use it more effectively.

Advances in technology have also enabled new ways of practicing hypnosis. Computer-assisted hypnosis and hypnosis apps are becoming increasingly popular, allowing people to access it in the comfort of their homes. These advances are democratizing access to hypnosis and offer new opportunities for its use in health care.

Beyond technology, hypnosis is finding new applications in a variety of fields. In sports medicine, it is being used to improve the performance and concentration of athletes. In education, hypnosis techniques are being explored to improve learning and memory. And in the field of dentistry, is changing the way we treat pain, anxiety and a host of other conditions.

Hypnodontics, in particular, is becoming an area of growing interest. Dentists are using hypnosis to help patients manage anxiety and fear, to control pain without the need for medication, and to improve recovery after procedures. As research continues to explore and validate these uses, it is likely that we will see an increase in the adoption of hypnosis in dental practice.

As we move into the 21st century, hypnosis is at an exciting crossroads. With the support of scientific research and the advancement of technology, this clinical tool is beginning to be recognized as a powerful and valid tool in medicine and psychology. However, much remains to be learned about how it works, how we can use it more effectively, and how it can change the way we deliver health care.

CHAPTER 2: FUNDAMENTALS OF HYPNOSIS

WHAT IS HYPNOSIS?

Hypnosis is a technique that involves the induction of an altered state of consciousness, known as trance, in which a person becomes more receptive to suggestions and has enhanced perception and memory (Heap, M., & Aravind, K. K., 2002). During this state, the person may concentrate intensely on a specific idea or image and may ignore other things (Kirsch, I., 1994). The key components of hypnosis include suggestion, relaxation, concentration and trance.

Suggestions are ideas or instructions given to the person during the trance state (Kirsch, I., 2000). These suggestions can be used to influence the person's thoughts, emotions and behaviors. For example, it may be suggested to feel a sense of relaxation and calmness, to experience a change in perception, such as a decrease in pain, or to perform a specific behavior, such as quitting smoking (Lynn, S. J., Kirsch, I., Barabasz, A., Cardeña, E., & Patterson, D., 2000).

Relaxation is often an important part of hypnosis, as it helps the person enter the trance state. Relaxation can involve physical relaxation, such as the release of muscle tension, and mental relaxation, such as the release of worry and stress (Hammond, D. C., 2010).

Concentration involves focusing attention on a specific idea or image and is a crucial component of hypnosis. During the trance state, the subject may concentrate intensely on a specific idea or image and may ignore other things (Rainville, P., Hofbauer, R. K., Bushnell, M. C., Duncan, G. H., & Price, D. D., 2002).

Trance is an altered state of consciousness in which a person becomes more receptive to suggestions and has enhanced perception and memory (Heap, M., & Aravind, K. K., 2002). During this state, the patient may focus intensely on a specific idea or image and may ignore other things.

Perhaps another way to understand hypnosis is from the way it is defined. Throughout history, hypnosis has been defined in different ways by various organizations and experts. The following are some of the most recognized definitions:

American Medical Association (AMA): In 1958, the AMA defined hypnosis as "a temporary state of altered attention in the individual, which may be induced by another person and in which a variety of phenomena may appear spontaneously or in response to verbal or nonverbal stimuli. These phenomena include changes in awareness and memory, increased susceptibility to suggestion, changes in sensory perception, feeling or behavior" (AMA, 1958).

The British Psychological Society (BPS): In its 2001 report, defines hypnosis as "a procedure during which one person, the hypnotist, suggests that another person, the subject, experience changes in sensations, perceptions, thoughts or behaviors" (BPS, 2001).

American Psychological Association (APA): On its website, the APA defines hypnosis as "a state of consciousness involving focused and reduced attention and increased receptivity to suggestion" (APA, n.d.).

Milton H. Erickson: Erickson, one of the most recognized pioneers in the field of hypnosis, defined hypnosis as "a special state of intrapersonal and interpersonal communication" (Erickson, 1980).

Importantly, although these definitions vary in their wording and approach, they all recognize that hypnosis involves a state of focused attention and increased receptivity to suggestions.

HOW HYPNOSIS WORKS

Hypnosis, despite having been studied for centuries, still retains some mystery as to its mechanism of action. Different theories seek to explain how hypnosis works, and the understanding of how it works has evolved over time. Here we explore several of these theories, from psychodynamic to cognitive and neuroscientific.

Dissociation theory

The theory of dissociation is one of the main theories explaining how hypnosis works. It was initially proposed by Pierre Janet and has been extended and elaborated by others, including Ernest Hilgard.

In Hilgard's model of dissociation, known as "neodissociation theory," it is argued that hypnosis creates a split in consciousness, which allows some things to occur in the mind without the primary consciousness being fully aware of them (Hilgard, 1977). The author suggested that hypnosis involves a separation between different aspects of consciousness, including awareness of the self and executive control processes.

For example, under hypnosis, a person could be directed not to feel pain in response to a painful stimulus. According to dissociation theory, the person's executive control system might recognize the stimulus as painful, but this recognition would be dissociated or separated from the consciousness of the self, so that the person would not experience the sensation of pain (Hilgard, 1977).

The dissociation theory has been supported by some research. For example, a 2017 study, in the journal Scientific Reports found evidence of dissociation in brain responses to painful stimuli during hypnosis (Jiang, White, Greicius, Waelde & Spie- gel, 2017).

Social role theory or role-demand theory

The social role theory is an alternative explanation for the phenomenon of hypnosis, proposed by Theodore R. Sarbin and William C. Coe. This theory suggests that hypnosis is essentially a social role that a person adopts, and not a special or altered state of consciousness.

According to Sarbin and Coe (1972), when a subject is hypnotized, he or she is assuming a role, similar to an actor in a play, and is acting in accordance with the expectations of that role. In the context of hypnosis, this involves meeting the hypnotist's and the subject's expectations about what he or she will yield during the treatment. For example, if hypnosis is expected to cause amnesia, the subject will act according to that expectation and "forget" what happened during the session.

This social role theory has had a significant influence on the field of hypnosis and has contributed to a shift in focus from hypnosis as an altered state of consciousness to an understanding of hypnosis in terms of expectations, beliefs, and social contexts.

Cognitive theory of hypnosis

The cognitive theory of hypnosis, proposed by Nicholas Spanos among others, suggests that the effects of hypnosis are the result of normal cognitive processes and expectations, rather than a special state of consciousness.

According to Spanos (1986), people in a state of hypnosis are not in an altered state of consciousness, but are playing a social role in which they are expected to follow the suggestions of the hypnotist. According to this theory, a person's ability to be hypnotized does not depend on a "special ability" or the capacity to enter an altered state of consciousness, but on his or her willingness to participate in the process and on his or her expectations and beliefs about what will happen during hypnosis.

Cognitive theory also holds that people in hypnosis process information differently than they normally would. Instead of analyzing and evaluating information critically, trance patients may accept the hypnotist's suggestions more literally and without question. This may allow them to experience changes in perception, memory and behavior that may not be possible in a normal state of consciousness.

Neuroscience of hypnosis

Neuroscience has made it possible to explore the impact of hypnosis on the brain. Neuroimaging techniques such as functional magnetic resonance imaging (fMRI) and electroencephalography (EEG) have shown changes in brain activity during hypnosis. For example, increased activity has been observed in areas of the brain related to attention and imagination, and decreased activity in areas related to self-criticism and self-awareness (Oakley & Halligan, 2013). These findings suggest that hypnosis may involve specific changes in brain function.

Despite the many theories, hypnosis is still not fully understood and is likely to involve a combination of psychological and neurophysiological factors. What is clear is that it can be a powerful tool for changing perception, thinking and behavior, and research continues to explore how and why this is so.

Clearly, there is great interest in understanding how it affects the brain, and as neuroimaging technologies advance, understanding of the mechanisms of action of hypnosis continues to evolve. However, the multifaceted nature of hypnosis means that it is unlikely that any single theory can explain it in its entirety. Rather, a combination of psychological, social, and neurophysiological factors interact to give rise to the unique experience that is hypnosis.

Hypnosis and the Default Mode Brain Network

Recent findings in neuroscience have provided a new approach to understanding how hypnosis works in the brain. In particular, the Default Mode Network (PMN), which includes brain regions that are activated when we are not focused on the outside world but absorbed in inner thoughts, may play an important role in hypnosis.

The MPN includes several brain regions that are activated during rest and introspection, and deactivated during tasks that require focused attention. According to Raichle et al. (2001), these brain areas are involved in functions such as self-reflection, imagination and internal narrative (Raichle 2001).

In the context of hypnosis, PMR may be relevant in several ways. Some investigators have suggested that during hypnosis, the therapist may be able to influence

The therapist may use the RMP to change the "story" that the subject tells himself about his experience, thus allowing for modification of perception and behavior. For example, a therapist might use hypnotic suggestion to help a subject imagine that his arm is anesthetized, which could change the subject's perception of the sensation in his arm.

PMR may also be involved in the "absorption" aspect of hypnosis. Some people are more able than others to engage deeply in imaginative experiences and to block out the outside world, a characteristic that is associated with the ability to be hypnotized. These people may have a particularly active or flexible PMR.

It is important to keep in mind that, although these findings are promising, research on the role of PMR in hypnosis is still in its early stages, and more studies are needed to fully understand these relationships.

Hypnosis and the Executive Control Network

The Executive Control Network (ECN) is a system of brain regions that play a central role in high-level cognitive tasks such as decision-making, attention, working memory and impulse control. Vincent et al. (2008) describe the ECN as an interconnected set of brain regions that work together to regulate our responses and behaviors, allowing us to react flexibly and adaptively to our environment.

In the context of hypnosis, the CER can play a particularly important role. During a hypnosis session, the connections between the ECN and other brain regions, as suggested by a study by McGeown et al. (2009). This may help explain why patients under hypnosis may show increased concentration and susceptibility to the hypnotist's suggestions. For example, CER could facilitate the focus of attention on the hypnotist's suggestions and help inhibit or block distractions.

In addition, CER may also be involved in how hypnosis can help people to modify their behavior or perception. Through hypnotic su- perception, the hypnotist can help the subject to imagine new ways of thinking or behaving, and the CER may play a role in the implementation and maintenance of these new patterns of thought or behavior.

However, as with many areas of hypnosis research, much remains to be learned about the exact role of the ECN and other brain networks in hypnosis. Further research and a better understanding of these brain networks could lead to new strategies and techniques to improve the effectiveness of hypnosis as a therapeutic tool.

PRINCIPLES OF HYPNOSIS

Understanding the fundamental principles behind hypnosis can help us understand how and why it works. The following are some of the key principles that facilitate hypnosis:

Focus of Attention

Focusing attention is one of the fundamental techniques in the practice of hypnosis, and has been considered one of the key underlying mechanisms for the onset of the hypnotic state. In simpler terms, it is the ability to direct and maintain attention to a specific focal point, often under the guidance of a hypnotist.

According to research, this focus of attention can have a number of psychological and physiological effects. From a psychological point of view, it can help per- sonnel block out distractions and focus on inner thoughts, feelings, or experiences (Raz & Li- fshitz, 2016). This can facilitate greater susceptibility to the hypnotist's suggestions, allowing more effective changes in behaviors, emotions, and thoughts to take place.

In addition, from a neurophysiological point of view, attentional focus has been shown to influence brain activity. Research has found that hypnosis can increase connectivity between the Executive Control Network (ECN) and other brain regions that are responsible for attention and cognitive control (McGeown et al., 2009). This could explain how hypnosis improves concentration and receptivity to suggestions.

However, not all people respond in the same way to hypnosis and some individuals may find easier than others to focus their attention. This may be related to a variety of factors, such as individual differences in the ability to focus, expectations about this therapeutic tool, and previous experiences of hypnosis.

Finally, it should be noted that attentional focus is a skill that can be improved with practice. Many hypnotists use training techniques and exercises to help people improve their ability to concentrate, which can increase the effectiveness of hypnosis.

Dissociation

Dissociation is a phenomenon that occurs when a person experiences a disconnection between his or her thoughts, memories, sensations, actions, or sense of identity. During hypnosis, dissociation can be a useful tool to help a person focus on his or her inner world and away from external distractions.

According to dissociation theory, hypnosis is viewed as a state in which conscious control of thought and action can be separated from consciousness (Hilgard, 1986). This may allow a person to concentrate intensely on a single task or thought, while his or her awareness of the external environment or the passage of time fades.

At a deeper level, dissociation may allow the separation of certain painful emotions or memories from immediate awareness. For example, a person under hypnosis may be able to recall a traumatic event without experiencing the emotional pain associated with it. This aspect of dissociation can be useful in trauma therapy, since that can enable patients to process painful experiences in a safe and controlled manner.

Dissociation can also be useful in pain control. By dissociating from physical sensations, a person may be able to experience physical pain without the emotional suffering normally associated with it. This use of dissociation can be useful in a variety of contexts, from chronic pain control to pain management during medical procedures.

It is important to note that although dissociation can be beneficial in hypnosis, it can also be a symptom of certain psychological disorders, such as posttraumatic stress disorder and other dissociative disorders. Therefore, it should be handled with care by trained professionals.

SUGGESTION AS A PRINCIPLE OF HYPNOSIS

Introduction to suggestion as a principle of hypnosis

Suggestion is a fundamental principle of hypnosis that plays a crucial role in the effectiveness of the practice. In hypnosis, suggestion refers to the commands or instructions given to subjects while they are in a trance state, which they are expected to carry out once they emerge from this altered state of consciousness. These suggestions are designed to create positive possibilities in the patient and generate minimal resistance. The process of suggestion is not limited to hypnosis alone, as it is also used by various entities, such as the media and books, to manipulate and influence people. The concept of suggestion has evolved over time, from its origins to the emergence of a more definite understanding of its capacity. Hypnosis itself is an altered state of consciousness, either self-induced or induced by another person, in which both psychological and physiological changes can be observed. Therefore, suggestion serves as a powerful tool for guiding and influencing the thoughts, feelings, and behaviors of people during hypnosis.

According to Hammond (2010), "Suggestion is one of the most important aspects of hypnosis, and is the key to its therapeutic effectiveness" . The importance of suggestion in hypnosis lies in its ability to guide the individual's experience and responses. Different types of suggestions can be used in hypnosis processes, each of which produces specific effects on the individual. Once a subject has reached the state of hypnosis, the suggestions can be tested to produce the desired effects.

by the hypnotist. These suggestions can be empowering and reinforcing, creating positive possibilities for the patient and generating minimal resistance. In the clinical field, hypnosis is often used, along with suggestion techniques, as a support tool for psychological therapeutic systems. The use of trance suggestion can help people overcome various challenges, such as controlling pain, reducing anxiety, or changing unwanted behaviors. The effectiveness of suggestion in hypnosis is based on the individual's receptivity and willingness to accept and act on the suggestions provided.

In conclusion, suggestion is a fundamental principle of hypnosis that plays a vital role in guiding and influencing people's thoughts, feelings and behaviors. It involves giving orders or instructions to subjects in a trance state, which they are expected to carry out once they regain their normal state of consciousness. Suggestion is not limited to hypnosis alone, as it is also used in various contexts to manipulate and influence people. The use of suggestion in hypnosis can have profound effects on people's mental and emotional well-being, enabling them to overcome challenges and make positive changes in their lives.

Types of suggestions used in hypnosis

There are different types of suggestions used in hypnosis to induce a desired state or behavior in people. One type is direct suggestions, where the hypnotist explicitly tells the individual what to do or experience. These suggestions are given in a precise and concise manner, often in a monotone, to enhance their effectiveness. Direct suggestions are straightforward and leave little room for interpretation.

According to Lynn and Green (2011), "Direct suggestions are those that specify the desired behavior or experience in clear and unambiguous terms" (p. 67). Another type of suggestion used in hypnosis is indirect suggestions. These are more subtle and can be delivered in a way that allows the individual to interpret and internalize the message. When indirect they often involve narratives, metaphors or hypothetical situations to influence the individual's subconscious mind. By bypassing the conscious mind, indirect suggestions can have a profound impact on beliefs, attitudes and behaviors.

Post-hypnotic suggestions are another important aspect of hypnosis. These suggestions are given during the hypnotic state, but are intended to be carried out after the individual has emerged from hypnosis. Post-hypnotic suggestions can be used to reinforce desired changes, such as breaking a habit or improving self-confidence. The individual may unconsciously perform actions or experience certain behaviors as a result of the post-hypnotic suggestion.

The power of suggestion to influence the behavior and beliefs

This power is a fundamental principle of hypnosis. Suggestions have the ability to alter perceptions and beliefs, both physically and psychologically. In the context of hypnosis, suggestions are used to guide people into a state of heightened suggestibility, where they are more receptive to accepting and acting on the suggestions provided. This process allows the potential for significant behavioral changes and transformations.

Examples of behavioral change through suggestion can be seen in various therapeutic applications of hypnosis. For example, it is often used to help people relax, reduce feelings of pain, or relieve anxiety. By harnessing the power of suggestion, hypnosis can facilitate these desired changes in subjective experiences and behaviors. In addition, cognitive-behavioral hypno- sis uses suggestion as a means of promoting behavioral change through the interaction between the hypnotist and the subject. These examples highlight the potential of suggestion to influence and shape behavior in a positive and constructive manner.

However, it is important to consider the ethical implications of the use of suggestions in hypnosis. While suggestions can be empowering and create positive possibilities for the individual, it is crucial to ensure that the suggestions are aligned with the individual's well-being and values. Ethical considerations should be taken into account to avoid misuse or manipulation of suggestions for personal gain, or to compel individuals to act against their own interests. By adhering to ethical guidelines, the power of suggestion in hypnosis can be harnessed responsibly and effectively for the benefit of patients seeking positive change.

The role of language and images in suggestion.

The use of language patterns is a crucial aspect of hypnotic suggestion. These patterns are designed to create empowering and reinforcing suggestions that generate minimal resistance in the patient. Hypnosis itself is a state of deep relaxation in which people are more open to suggestion, allowing for modifications in beliefs and behavioral patterns.

According to Heap and Aravind (2002), "Language is the primary tool for the hypnotist and, therefore, it is important that effective language patterns are used to achieve the desired results". The renowned psychiatrist and hypnotherapist Milton Erickson developed principles and strategies based on these language patterns, which have been widely used in the field of hypnosis. By carefully choosing and structuring their words, hypnotherapists can effectively guide people toward positive possibilities and desired outcomes.

The creation of vivid imagery is another key element in the suggestion process during hypnosis. The use of visual imagery helps to capture the patient's attention and enhances the effectiveness of the suggestions provided. Hypnotherapists employ techniques such as modulation of suggestion wording, including pacing, voice inflections, and key terms, to create a more engaging and impactful experience for the individual.

According to Yapko (2012), "Visual suggestion is a common technique in hypnosis, which involves transforming the desired outcome into a mental image, further reinforcing the suggestions made through verbal communication." By incorporating vivid imagery into hypnotic suggestions, hypnotherapists can harness the power of the subconscious mind and facilitate positive changes in behavior and perception.

In conclusion, the impact of language and imagery on suggestibility is significant. Although hypnosis allows people to be more receptive to suggestions, it is important to note that no one can be induced to accept suggestions that go against his or her ethical and moral principles. The aim of certain behavioral programs is to increase receptivity to suggestions from non-hypnotic subjects.

suggestive. Suggestion has been an integral part of human communication since ancient times and has evolved into the practice of hypnosis. In the field of sports psychology, the efficacy of hypnosis has been recognized in the use of suggestion techniques as an adjunct to therapeutic systems. In general, the use of language and imagery in suggestion plays a vital role in harnessing the power of the mind and facilitating positive change in people.

Improving suggestibility through relaxation and focus

Relaxation plays a crucial role in the hypnosis process. By inducing a state of deep laxity, people become more open and receptive to suggestions. This state of relaxation allows the conscious mind to quiet down, making it easier for the hypnotist to access the subconscious mind and introduce positive suggestions. The use of relaxation techniques in hypnosis has been found to be effective in reducing anxiety and increasing control over emotions. In addition, relaxation helps to relieve tension in the body, allowing people to enter a receptive and centered state, which is essential for successful hypnosis.

Techniques for inducing relaxation in hypnosis vary, but often involve progressive muscle relaxation, deep breathing exercises, and guided imagery. Progressive muscle relaxation, for example, involves systematically tensing and relaxing different muscle groups of the body, promoting a state of physical and mental laxity. Deep breathing exercises help people to slow down their breathing, promoting a sense of calmness and relaxation [30]. Guided imagery involves visualizing peaceful and serene scenes, which enables people mentally escape and enter a state of relaxation. These techniques can be used individually or in combination to help induce a state of deep relaxation, enhancing suggestibility during the hypnotic process.

In addition to relaxation, hypnosis aims to increase focus and receptivity to suggestions. By directing the individual's attention and focus, the hypnotist can bypass the critical conscious mind and communicate directly with the subconscious mind. This increased focus allows people to become more receptive to positive suggestions, such as changing behaviors or overcoming challenges. Studies have shown that hypnosis can be effective in increasing self-efficacy and reducing negative affect. By harnessing the power of suggestion and improving focus, hypnosis can be a powerful tool for personal growth and self-improvement.

Overcoming resistance to suggestion

This is a crucial aspect of effective hypnosis utilization. In the clinical setting, the hypnotist relies on his or her communication skills to guide clients to accept suggestions. However, resistance to suggestion can be a challenge.

On the other hand, Lynn and Green (2011), state that "Resistance to suggestion can be an obstacle to successful hypnosis, and it is important that the hypnotist understands the common barriers to suggestion and has strategies to overcome them." To overcome resistance, it is essential to iden- tify the common barriers to suggestion. These barriers may include skepticism, fear, and lack of trust in the hypnotist or the process itself. By understanding these barriers, hypnotists can adapt their approach to address and overcome them.

Strategies to overcome this resistance in hypnosis involve several techniques. According to Heap and Aravind (2002), "A positive and supportive therapeutic relationship is crucial for enhancing suggestibility." By establishing a positive and supportive therapeutic relationship, hypnotists can create an environment in which clients feel comfortable and open to suggestions. In addition, restructuring resistance in the form of suggestion can be an efficacious approach. Skilled hypnotists reframe resistance, presenting it as an opportunity for positive change and transformation. Indirect suggestions, such as parables and metaphors, can also be used to bypass the conscious mind and access the subconscious.

The use of suggestion hypnosis has been studied and applied in various therapeutic contexts. According to Barabasz and Barabasz (2006), "Hypnosis with suggestion has been shown to be particularly effective in controlling anxiety and improving confidence in athletes". By utilizing suggestive techniques, hypnosis can assist in therapeutic systems, helping individuals to overcome challenges and achieve positive outcomes. The development of therapeutic skills and techniques in hypnosis is crucial to increasing confidence in therapy and teaching self-hypnosis. Understanding the historical evolution of hypnosis and its connection to its management provides a contextual framework for its application. In general, suggestion remains a fundamental principle of hypnosis, enabling people to overcome resistance and achieve positive change.

Use of suggestion for therapeutic purposes

Suggestion is a fundamental principle in the practice of hypnosis, particularly in therapeutic settings. Its application in therapy involves using verbal cues and techniques to influence thoughts, behaviors, and behaviors of the patient.

and emotions of a person. Hypnosis, often used in conjunction with suggestion, allows people to enter a relaxed state of heightened suggestibility, making them more receptive to therapeutic interventions. In clinical hypnosis, suggestion techniques are used as an aid in various therapeutic systems. These suggestions are designed to enhance and reinforce positive possibilities in the patient, generating favorable results. Their use in therapy has gained great interest and recognition in recent years.

There are numerous examples of therapeutic interventions that incorporate suggestion techniques. One example is the use of therapeutic hypnosis, also known as clinical hypnosis, which aims to combat automated suggestions, programs or operations that may be causing distress or negative behaviors. Another example is the use of suggestion in catharsis, where the therapist guides the patient to express thoughts and emotions, facilitating a healthy release of ideas. These interventions highlight the power of suggestion to promote positive changes in people and facilitate therapeutic progress.

Research has been conducted to explore their efficacy in therapy. Studies have shown that hypnosis and suggestion can elicit specific responses in the brain, activating specific areas associated with hypnotic phenomena. The therapeutic efficacy of hypnosis, particularly in the form of directed suggestion, has been recognized as a valid field of study. In addition, the use of suggestion techniques, such as hypnosis, has been shown to be effective in the teaching-learning process. These findings further highlight the importance and potential benefits of using it in therapeutic interventions.

Conclusion: Harnessing the Power of Suggestion in Hypnosis

The principle of suggestion plays a vital role in hypnosis, as it involves potentiating and reinforcing suggestions that create positive possibilities in the patient. Suggestion has been a fundamental component of hypnosis since its inception. In fact, as early as 1888, hypnotic suggestion was used to eliminate patient suffering. Over time its use has evolved and expanded, and practitioners recognize its importance in facilitating positive change. Even Sigmund Freud, a leading figure in the field of psychology, recognized the power of suggestion in the doctor-patient relationship. Thus, suggestion serves as the cornerstone of hypnosis, allowing people to access their subconscious mind and explore new possibilities for personal growth and healing.

The benefits of using it in hypnosis are numerous. Hypnotherapy, which incorporates suggestion-based techniques, has been shown to be effective in the treatment of a variety of conditions, such as sleep problems, bedwetting, smoking cessation, and eating disorders. In addition, suggestion can be used in cognitive restructuring, particularly in the treatment of addictions. However, it is important to recognize the limitations of suggestion-based hypnosis. While it may be effective for many people, not everyone responds equally to suggestion and results may vary. In addition, the success of suggestion-based hypnosis relies on the skill and experience of the hypnotherapist to provide personalized suggestions that resonate with the individual's subconscious mind. Nevertheless, the potential benefits of suggestion-based hypnosis make it a valuable tool in the field of therapeutic interventions.

As the field of hypnosis continues to advance, there are ongoing efforts to explore new directions and advances in suggestion-based hypnosis. Specialists are investigating the use of hypnosis and suggestion in the teaching-learning process, recognizing its potential to enhance learning and performance. In addition, the integration of technology, such as virtual reality, may offer new opportunities for using suggestion. By harnessing the power of suggestion and incorporating innovative approaches, the field of hypnosis can continue to evolve and expand its potential to promote personal growth, healing, and wellness.

RELAXATION AS A PRINCIPLE OF HYPNOSIS

Introduction

Relaxation is a fundamental principle of hypnosis and plays a crucial role in the induction of a hypnotic state. In the context of hypnosis, relaxation refers to the process of achieving a state of deep physical and mental calm, which allows the individual to enter a heightened state of suggestibility (Hammond, 1990). While it is important to keep in mind that hypnosis is not only about relaxation, as unconscious processes also occur, the state of physical and mental calm serves as a fundamental component in facilitating the hypnotic experience (Kirsch, 1994). The inclusion of relaxation techniques in hypnosis sessions aims to promote a sense of calmness, well-being and receptivity to suggestions (Yapko, 2012). This principle is emphasized in several training programs, such as the Master's Degree in Clinical Hypnosis and Relaxation (University of Salamanca, 2021), where psychologists learn to induce hypnosis by helping their patients to relax in real time.

The induction phase of hypnosis focuses on freeing the conscious mind and opening the subconscious, preparing the individual for deep rest (Erickson, Rossi & Rossi, 1976). By inducing a change in the state of consciousness and increasing relaxation, hypnosis improves attention and concentration, making the individual more receptive to therapeutic suggestions (Hammond, 1990). Research by Hernández Mendo et al. (2003) highlights that hypnosis can be activated and invoked spontaneously, with induction methods taking different forms, including calming and relaxation. In addition, during hypnotic induction, suggestions can be adapted to the respiratory rhythm.

of the patient, promoting a seamless integration of relaxation and unconscious receptivity (Banyai, Hilgard & Johnson, 1964). Therefore, physical and mental calmness serves as a vital component in facilitating the hypnotic state and optimizing the effectiveness of hypnosis (Hammond, 1990).

The use of hypnosis for relaxation and subconscious suggestion has been well established for over a century (Erickson, Rossi & Rossi, 1976). While there may be debate about the need for relaxation to achieve certain hypnotic drivers and subjective changes, it remains a common and widely used element in hypnosis sessions (Lynn, Kirsch & Hallquist, 2008). In fact, each hypnosis session usually includes an initial or preparatory phase in which the patient is guided to relax and induce a calm state (Spiegel, 1993). The relaxation aspect of hypnosis not only contributes to the overall experience, but also has the potential to reduce stress, provide positive feedback, and eliminate negative thoughts (Wickramasekera II, 2001). By incorporating these techniques, hypnosis offers individuals the opportunity to achieve deep calm and access their subconscious mind for therapeutic purposes.

Understand the physiological and physiological aspects of
psychological aspects of relaxation

Relaxation plays a crucial role in the practice of hypnosis, as it is both a physiological and a psychological principle. Physiologically, deep tranquility induces several changes in the body, such as a decrease in heart rate, blood pressure, and muscle tension. These changes are essential for entering a state of deep relaxation, which is a prerequisite for successful hypnosis. By promoting calmness, hypnosis enables people to achieve a greater state of mindfulness and relaxation.

concentration, which allows them to respond better to therapeutic suggestions and interventions (Hammond, 1990). Thus, relaxation serves as the basis for the hypnotic experience, facilitating a deeper level of engagement and receptivity.

In addition to its physiological effects, relaxation also offers numerous psychological benefits. Practicing relaxation techniques can help people reduce stress and anxiety, promoting a sense of calm and well-being (Wickramasekera II, 2001). It has been found to improve sleep quality, help control insomnia and promote restful sleep (Lichstein et al., 2006). In addition, relaxation techniques can improve concentration, memory, and cognitive functioning, allowing individuals to better manage their daily tasks and responsibilities (Elliott et al., 2014). By incorporating relaxation into their daily routine, individuals may experience greater mental clarity, emotional stability, and overall psychological well-being (Jain et al., 2007).

The role of relaxation in reducing stress and anxiety is particularly important. Hypnosis can be an effective tool for managing and relieving stress and anxiety (Hammond, 1990). By inducing a state of deep relaxation, hypnosis helps people access their subconscious mind and reframe negative thought patterns and beliefs (Yapko, 2012). This can lead to a reduction in anxiety symptoms and an increased sense of calm and relaxation. In addition, relaxation techniques used in conjunction with hypnosis can enhance the effectiveness of stress and anxiety management strategies (Schoenberger et al., 2002). By promoting it, hypnosis provides individuals with a valuable tool for coping with the challenges of daily life and promoting their overall well-being.

Techniques to induce relaxation in hypnosis

One of the key principles of hypnosis is to induce relaxation in the individual. There are various techniques that can be used to achieve this state. One of these techniques is progressive muscle relaxation, which was devised by Edmund Jacobson at the beginning of the 20th century (Jacobson, 1929). Progressive muscle relaxation consists of tensing and then relaxing different muscle groups of the body, leading to a deep state of laxity (Jacobson, 1938). This technique has been found to be effective in relieving pain, improving sleep and promoting general mental calmness (Bernstein & Borkovec, 1973).

Another technique to induce relaxation in hypnosis is deep breathing exercises. Pro- found breathing is a powerful tool to reduce stress and promote relaxation in the body (Brown & Gerbarg, 2005). When we breathe deeply, our body sends signals to the brain to activate the relaxation response, leading to a decrease in heart rate and blood pressure (Brown & Gerbarg, 2012). Deep breathing exercises can be practiced in a variety of ways, such as diaphragmatic breathing or ab- dominal breathing, where the breath is inhaled deeply into the abdomen (Stanciu, 2015). By incorporating deep breathing techniques into hypnosis sessions, people can experience a greater sense of relaxation and inner peace.

Guided imagery and visualization are also techniques commonly used to induce relaxation in hypnosis. Guided imagery involves the creation of vivid mental images and scenarios that promote a sense of relaxation and calm (Rossman, 2002). By guiding

Through a visualization process, people can imagine themselves in peaceful and calm environments, allowing their mind and body to relax (Naparstek, 2000). Guided imagery has been shown to be effective in reducing stress, anxiety and promoting general well-being (Best, 2010). It can be particularly beneficial for people who find it difficult to visualize, as it provides a structured framework for relaxation (Holmes & Burish, 1981). Incorporating guided imagery into hypnosis sessions can help people achieve a deep state of laxity and harness their subconscious mind for positive change (Hammond, 1990).

The importance of creating a relaxed environment for hypnosis

Creating a relaxed environment is a crucial principle in the practice of hypnosis. The environment in which hypnosis takes place must be conducive to relaxation and reduction of disturbing stimuli (Hammond, 2010). This includes establishing the appropriate environment, whether it is a comfortable room or a specific chair or bed that promotes relaxation (Lynn & Kirsch, 2006). By creating a calm and peaceful atmosphere, people are more likely to enter a state of deep relaxation, which is essential for successful hypnosis (Spiegel, 1993). The ability to induce oneself into a state of deep relaxation or self-hypnosis is also a valuable skill to develop (Hammond, 2000).

Eliminating distractions is another important aspect of creating a relaxed environment for hypnosis. Dis- tractions can disrupt the individual's focus and hinder his or her ability to enter a relaxed state (Heap, Brown & Oakley, 2010). Therefore, it is essential to minimize or eliminate any possible source of distraction, such as turning off electronic devices or ensuring that the space is quiet and undisturbed (Elkins et al., 2015). This allows people to fully participate in the hypnotic process and enhance their receptivity to the su- gestions (Tinterow, 1999).

The use of music or soothing sounds can also contribute to the relaxation process during hypnosis. Music has the power to evoke emotions and create an ideal atmosphere. Certain types of music, such as spa music or nature sounds, are specifically designed to induce relaxation and promote a sense of calm (Kwekkeboom et al., 2012). Listening to relaxing music can help people enter a state of deep calm and enhance their general hypnotic experience (Kwekkeboom, Wanta & Bumpus, 2008). In addition, binaural sounds, which involve hearing different frequencies in each ear, have been found to stimulate positive ac- titude and aid the process (Padmanabhan, Hildreth & Laws 2010). By incorporating these auditory elements into the hypnosis session, practitioners can further facilitate relaxation and create a more conducive environment for hypnosis practice (Hammond, 2010).

The role of relaxation in accessing the subconscious mind

Relaxation plays a crucial role in the practice of hypnosis, particularly when it comes to accessing the subconscious mind. According to Lynn and Green (2011), "Relaxation is an important component in hypnosis, as it allows people to bypass the conscious mind and access deeper levels of awareness." By inducing a state of relaxation, hypnosis allows people to bypass the conscious mind and access deeper levels of consciousness. This is important because the mind

The conscious mind often filters and analyzes information, making it difficult to access and work with the subconscious mind. Through relaxation, the conscious mind becomes less active, allowing the subconscious mind to come to the forefront.

In addition to bypassing the conscious mind, calmness also increases an individual's suggestibility during hypnosis. According to Spiegel and Greenleaf (2005), "Relaxation is a fundamental tool in hypnosis, as it reduces the conscious mind's ability to filter or question hypnotic suggestions." When the mind and body are in a relaxed state, they become more open and receptive to suggestions. This heightened state of suggestibility allows the hypnotist to effectively communicate with the subconscious mind and implant positive suggestions or beliefs.

According to Shenefelt (2010), "Relaxation is a fundamental component of hypnosis for anxiety control, as it can help reduce the physical and mental tension associated with anxiety". Thus, relaxation not only facilitates access to the subconscious mind but also enhances the power of hypnotic suggestions.

In addition, relaxation techniques are used to enhance the hypnotic state and improve the overall effectiveness of hypnosis. According to Heap and Aravind (2002), "Relaxation is the basis of many hypnosis techniques, as it is essential for inducing a deep hypnotic state." Techniques such as progressive relaxation, developed by Edmund Jacobson, focus on systematically loosening the body and mind. By achieving a deep state of relaxation, the individual becomes more receptive to the hypnotic process and the suggestions given by the hypnotist.

In general, relaxation serves as a fundamental principle in hypnosis, allowing people to access their subconscious mind and experience the transformative power of suggestion.

The relationship between relaxation and trance states

Relaxation plays a crucial role in inducing a trance state during hypnosis. Hypnosis itself is an altered state of consciousness, either self-induced or induced by a hypnotist, and relaxation is often used as the primary method to facilitate the induction process. By guiding people into a state of deep relaxation, the conscious mind becomes more receptive to suggestions, allowing the subconscious mind to open and become more accessible. The induction process serves to free the conscious mind and prepare the person to relax deeply, creating the foundation for a trance state to occur. Thus, relaxation acts as a gateway to the hypnotic state and establishes a connection with the subconscious mind.

Deepening the state of relaxation is an essential aspect of promoting trance during hypnosis. As people become more relaxed, their bodies may enter a cataleptic state or medium trance, where they experience a deep sense of physical and mental laxity. In this state, people may exhibit a total rigidity or complete abandonment of their bodies, allowing for a greater level of receptivity to hypnotic suggestions. Therapists use various techniques to adjust and deepen the state of relaxation, ensuring that people maintain the desired trance state throughout the session. Deepening the state of relaxation enhances the effectiveness of hypnosis by allowing a greater focus of attention.

and concentration. This heightened state of calm allows people to access their subconscious mind more easily and participate in the therapeutic work.

Achieving a deep state of relaxation during hypnosis offers numerous benefits for individuals. Research has found that hypnosis can reduce pain, including cancer-related pain and labor pain, as well as relieve symptoms such as nausea and vomiting. In addition, hypnosis can be used to address a variety of psychological problems, such as anxiety, phobias and smoking cessation. By inducing a deep state of relaxation, people can experience a sense of calm and inner peace, leading to greater overall well-being. The Master's Degree in Clinical Hypnosis and Relaxation aims to equip psychologists with the necessary skills to effectively use hypnosis and relaxation techniques in real-time clinical settings, further highlighting the importance of relaxation in the practice of hypnosis. In general, relaxation serves as a fundamental principle of hypnotism, allowing people to access their subconscious mind and work toward positive change and healing.

Potential challenges to achieving relaxation during hypnosis

Achieving relaxation during hypnosis can pose potential challenges for both the hypnotist and the hypnotized individual. A common challenge is dealing with resistance to relaxation. Some people may have difficulty letting go and allowing themselves to relax completely. This resistance can stem from a number of factors, such as fear of losing control or lack of trust in the hypnotist. Overcoming this resistance requires building rapport and trust with the individual, as well as addressing any concerns or misconceptions you may have about hypnosis.

Another challenge to achieving relaxation during hypnosis is addressing anxiety or fear related to the relaxation process itself. Some people may experience anxiety or fear when entering a deep state of calm because they may feel unfamiliar or uncomfortable. In such cases, it is important for the hypnotist to create a safe and supportive environment, reassuring the person that he or she is in control and that relaxation is a natural and beneficial state. By addressing and alleviating these anxieties, the individual can more easily calm down and participate fully in the hypnotic process.

Distractions can also make it difficult to relax during hypnosis. In today's fast-paced, technology-driven world, it can be a challenge for people to disconnect from external stimuli and fully immerse themselves in the hypnotic experience. The hypnotist must create a distraction-free environment, ensuring that the individual feels comfortable and can concentrate solely on the techniques being used. This may involve minimizing external noise, dimming the lights and providing guidance on how to put aside any racing thoughts or worries. By overcoming distractions, the individual can achieve a deeper state of tranquility, enhancing the effectiveness of the hypnosis session.

The hypnotist's role in facilitating relaxation

The hypnotist's role in facilitating relaxation is crucial in the hypnosis process. To generate this state, the hypnotist must first establish rapport and trust with the client. This creates a safe and comfortable environment for the client to relax and let go. The hypnotist can engage the client in conversation, actively listening and show empathy to build a strong therapeutic alliance. By creating a trusting relationship, the hypnotist can help the client feel comfortable and more receptive to relaxation suggestions.

Language and tone play an important role in the induction of relaxation during hypnosis. The hypnotist uses soothing and comforting language, along with a soft tone of voice, to guide the client into a state of deep relaxation. By using words and phrases that promote relaxation, such as "letting go," "deep breaths," and "feeling calm," the hypnotist helps the client enter a relaxed state of mind. The hypnotist's language and tone are carefully chosen to create a sense of comfort and security, allowing the client to release tension and reach a state of calmness.

Throughout the process, the hypnotherapist or dentist provides guidance and support to the client. This may involve giving instructions on deep breathing, progressive muscle relaxation or visualization techniques. The hypnotist may also use imagery and storytelling to engage the client's imagination and further enhance the experience. By offering guidance and support, the hypnotist helps the client move through the relaxation process and deepen the client's state. This creates an optimal environment for the client to experience the benefits of hypnosis, such as stress reduction and increased concentration.

The long-term benefits of incorporating the relaxation in hypnosis sessions

Incorporating relaxation techniques into hypnosis sessions can have long-term benefits for individuals. One of the main advantages is a greater sense of relaxation in daily life. By practicing it during hypnosis, people can learn to bring about a state of calm and tranquility more easily, which can then be applied to various situations outside hypnosis. Jacobson's method, for example, focuses on the principle that mental relaxation accompanies the absence of muscular contraction. While it is possible to undergo hypnosis without being in a relaxed state, laxity of both body and mind is a characteristic that most people associate with hypnosis. Therefore, incorporating relaxation techniques into hypnosis sessions can help people experience a greater sense of peace in their daily lives.

Another benefit of incorporating relaxation into hypnosis sessions is to improve sleep and overall well-being. When it is deep, achieved through hypnosis, it can help people achieve a state of calmness that promotes better sleep. Studies have shown that hypnosis can be a natural solution for improving sleep and managing sleep disorders. By inducing a state of deep relaxation, hypnosis can help people experience more restful and rejuvenating sleep, leading to better overall well-being.

Conclusion

In conclusion, relaxation is a fundamental principle of hypnosis that plays a crucial role in its effectiveness. Hypnosis consists of inducing a state of increased relaxation and

This state of relaxation creates an environment conducive for the therapist to guide the individual toward the desired goals. This state of relaxation creates an environment conducive for the therapist to guide the individual toward the desired goals. Early pioneers of hypnosis, such as James Braid, recognized the importance of relaxation in practice and emphasized the need for the patient to be in a relaxed state. The initial phase of a hypnosis session focuses on helping the patient relax and enter a receptive state. By incorporating relaxation techniques into hypnosis, therapists can effectively address stress-related problems and promote overall well-being. Thus, relaxation serves as the foundation for the success of hypnosis as a therapeutic tool.

It is important that hypnosis practitioners recognize the importance of relaxation and actively incorporate relaxation techniques into their practice. By using guided relaxation techniques, therapists can help their clients achieve a deep state of relaxation, which is essential for the induction of hypnosis. By incorporating relaxation techniques, therapists can improve the overall effectiveness of their hypnosis sessions and improve client outcomes. It is crucial that therapists continually explore and refine their understanding and application of relaxation techniques in the context of hypnosis. This ongoing exploration will contribute to the development of more effective and personalized hypnosis approaches that can benefit individuals seeking therapeutic intervention.

RAPPORT

Introduction to rapport in hypnosis

Rapport plays a crucial role in the practice of hypnosis, serving as a fundamental principle for establishing a hypnotic connection between the hypnotist and the subject. In hypnosis, rapport refers to the harmonious and trusting relationship between the two parties involved, characterized by empathy, understanding and effective communication. Hypnosis itself is an altered state of consciousness, either self-induced or induced by a hypnotist, where psychological and physiological changes can be observed. The establishment of a relationship is essential to create a safe and conducive environment for the hypnotic process to take place. It allows the subject to feel comfortable, trust the hypnotist and be more receptive to the suggestions and guidance given during the session.

Yapko, M. D. (2003) in his book "Trancework: An Intro- duction to the Practice of Clinical Hypnosis" discusses at length the importance of rapport in hypnosis and offers tips and strategies for building and maintaining an effective rapport with clients.

Building rapport through nonverbal communication is a crucial aspect of establishing a successful hypnotic connection with the client. According to Heap and Aravind (2002), "In any therapeutic process, including hypnosis, it is critical to create an environment of empathy, trust, and warmth to facilitate the hypnotic process." Non-verbal cues, such as body language, play an important role in creating a sense of trust, empathy, and understanding between hypnotist and client. The relationship is achieved by aligning verbal language, body language and emotional language.

Matching and mirroring techniques are commonly used to build rapport through nonverbal communication. According to Lynn and Green (2011), "These techniques involve subtly mimicking the client's body language, gestures, and posture to establish a sense of cone- xion and similarity." By matching and mirroring the patient's nonverbal cues, the hypnotist can create a subconscious bond, leading to greater rapport and trust.

Eye contact and facial expressions also play a crucial role in building rapport during hypnosis. According to Lynn and Green (2011), "Maintaining appropriate eye contact conveys attention, interest, and sincerity, which are essential for establishing trust and rapport." By maintaining consistent eye contact, the hypnotist demonstrates presence and engagement in the therapeutic process, fostering a sense of connection and understanding with the subject. In addition, facial expressions, such as smiling or nodding, can further enhance the relationship by conveying empathy and positive reinforcement.

In general, nonverbal communication plays an important role in building a strong and effective rapport during hypnosis. By paying attention to and effectively using nonverbal cues, a hypnotist can establish a strong rapport with the client, enhancing the effectiveness of the hypnotic session.

Establishing a relationship through verbal communication

Establishing rapport through verbal communication is a crucial aspect of hypnosis. One way to build rapport is through active listening skills. Active listening involves concentrating on and fully understanding what the other person is saying, without interrupting or judging.

By actively listening to the client's words, tone and body language, the hypnotist can demonstrate genuine interest and create a sense of trust and connection. This helps establish a safe and comfortable environment for the client, allowing them to open up and participate more deeply in the hypnotic process.

Empathy and understanding are also key components in establishing a relationship in hypnosis. Empathy involves putting oneself in the client's shoes, understanding their emotions, and showing them that their experiences are valid and understood. By demonstrating empathy, the hypnotist can create a sense of validation and support, which further strengthens the relationship between them and the client. This allows the patient to feel heard and understood, leading to a deeper level of trust and cooperation during the hypnosis session.

Language patterns play an important role in establishing rapport in hypnosis. Using language that is congruent with the individual's beliefs, values, and experiences can help create a sense of familiarity and connection. This can be achieved by mirroring the client's speech patterns, pacing the client's speech, and using similar vocabulary. In doing so, the hypnotist establishes a sense of rapport and resonance with the patient, making it easier to guide the patient into a hypnotic state and facilitate positive change.

Create a positive and trusting environment

This environment is crucial for establishing rapport during hypnosis, which can facilitate positive change in the client. According to Kohen (2008), "Rapport is one of the most important factors in the success of hypnosis." The first step in setting the stage for the building of a good relationship is to create a safe and comfortable space for the client. By creating this environment the client will feel at ease and more open to the hypnotic process.

Fostering trust and rapport through authenticity and sincerity is another important aspect of building a positive therapeutic relationship. According to Lynn and Green (2011), "The therapist should strive to be genuine and transparent, demonstrating authenticity in his or her words and actions." When clients perceive the therapist to be sincere, they are more likely to feel comfortable and trust the hypnosis process. By building trust and rapport, the therapist can create a supportive and collaborative partnership with the client, enhancing the effectiveness of the hypnotic experience.

The principles of relationship building in hypnosis are deeply rooted in the work of the renowned hypnotherapist Milton H. Erickson. According to Yapko (2012), "Erickson emphasized the importance of establishing rapport with clients as a means of facilitating positive change." By creating a positive and con- fidence-building environment through rapport building, the therapist can enhance receptivity to suggestions and increase the likelihood of achieving desired outcomes.

In general, rapport serves as a foundational principle of hypnosis, allowing the therapist to establish a strong therapeutic alliance and facilitate transformative change in the individual.

Build a relationship with different personality types.

Adaptation of communication style and relationship-building techniques are critical to the success of the project.

establishing a good rapport during hypnosis, especially when working with people of different personality types. According to Lynn and Green (2011), "The relationship between hypnotist and patient is crucial in hypnosis, and a personalized approach to relationship building can enhance the effectiveness of the hypnotic session."

Adapting to different communication styles allows the hypnotist to establish trust and understanding, which are essential for effective hypnosis. According to Eimer (2010), "The hypnotist must pay attention to the client's verbal and nonverbal cues to adapt to his or her communication style." In doing so, the hypnotist can create a more receptive environment for hypnosis.

Recognizing and responding to individual preferences is also important for establishing rapport and improving the effectiveness of hypnotic suggestions. According to Kohen (2008), "The hypnotist should tailor his or her suggestions and language to align with the individual's preferred style." By doing so, the hypnotist can create a more personalized and impactful hypnosis experience.

Adjusting relationship-building techniques for introverts and extroverts is another important aspect of working with different personality types. According to Lynn and Green (2011), "When establishing a relationship with introverts, it is important to create a calm and comfortable environment that allows them to feel safe and secure." On the other hand, when working with extroverts, engaging in more interactive and dynamic relationship-building activities can be effective. By tailoring techniques to sa- tisfy the preferences of introverts and extroverts, the hypnotist can establish a stronger connection and facilitate a more successful hypnosis session.

Maintaining and deepening the relationship along of the hypnotic process

Maintaining and deepening the relationship is a crucial principle in the practice of hypnosis. Continuous monitoring of rapport is essential to ensure a strong connection between hypnotist and patient throughout the hypnotic process. By paying attention to verbal and nonverbal cues, the hypnotist can gauge the level of rapport and make the necessary adjustments to tailor his or her techniques to individual needs and preferences.

Adapting techniques as needed is another important aspect of maintaining rapport in hypnosis. Each individual is unique, and what works for one client may not work for another. The hypnotist must be flexible and willing to modify his or her approach to suit each client's specific circumstances and personality. In doing so, the hypnotist can ensure that the client feels understood and supported, which strengthens the relationship between them.

This positive reinforcement and validation is a powerful way to deepen the connection between hypnotist and client. Positive reinforcement and validation of the client's progress and efforts can increase the client's confidence and motivation. This encourages the client to continue to participate in the hypnotic process and increases his or her trust in the hypnotist. By constantly reinforcing the relationship, the hypnotist creates a safe and supportive environment, which enhances the effectiveness of the hypnosis sessions.

The importance of therapeutic rapport has also been highlighted by research. According to Martin, Garske and Da- vis (2000), therapeutic rapport has a moderate but significant effect on therapy outcomes. Therefore, maintaining and deepening the relationship is essential to ensure the success of the hypnotic process.

THE EXPECTATION

Introduction to the principle of expectation in hypnosis

Kirsch, I. (1997), in his "Expectation Response Model," has argued that hypnosis is a form of suggestion influenced by the person's expectations and beliefs. According to Kirsch, the greater the expectation that something will happen, the more likely it is to happen, especially in the context of hypnosis.

This principle plays a crucial role in the practice of hypnosis. In the context of hypnosis, expectancy refers to the anticipation of a specific outcome or response. It is based on the concept of response expectancy, which is the belief or anticipation of an automatic reaction. Expectancy is a fundamental element in inducing a trance state during hypnosis. When people have a strong expectation of entering trance and experiencing the suggested effects, they are more likely to reach a hypnotic state. The response expectancy hypothesis, developed within the social-psychological or cognitive-behavioral perspective of hypnosis, emphasizes its importance in the process. This principle is exemplified in the case of Victor Rase, a patient who demonstrated superior knowledge and skills during a trance state, despite the fact that he did not remember upon awakening. Thus, expectancy serves as a key factor in facilitating the induction of a hypnotic state.

It also plays an important role in achieving the desired results through hypnosis. While the results of hypnosis are still being

By studying the exact mechanisms underlying hypnosis and its effects, research has shown that response expectancy is a variable that influences hypnotic behavior. Positive expectancies can enhance the effectiveness of hypnosis in helping people cope with pain, stress, and anxiety. Its power is further emphasized in studies that have explored the placebo effect, which is based on the belief and expectation of a positive outcome. In the context of hypnosis, creating positive expectations in the individual can lead to favorable outcomes and results. Therefore, this principle in hypnosis is crucial to achieve the desired therapeutic goals and outcomes.

The principle of expectancy in hypnosis has been the subject of research and exploration in the field of psychotherapy. Hypnosis has played a prominent role in the development of several schools of psychotherapy, as it provides a scientific explanation of the role of expectancy in inducing therapeutic change. Research on response expectancy as a variable underlying hypnotic behavior has contributed to a deeper understanding of the mechanisms at play. In addition, its importance as a motivational factor in hypnosis has been recognized, as it encourages people to enter a trance state and participate in the therapeutic process. Therefore, this principle is important both in terms of its practical application and its contribution to the theoretical understanding of the field.

The power of suggestion and its connection to expectation

Suggestion is a fundamental technique used in hypnosis to create positive expectations in the hypnotic subject. One of the most effective techniques is the use of imagery.

vivid and detailed. By presenting these images to the subject through suggestion, the hypnotist can evoke powerful sensory experiences and enhance the subject's hopes for the suggested outcome." (Kihlstrom, 2008)

Suggestion has the ability to influence the mind and create expectations in the hypnotic subject. Suggestion can be defined as the process of communicating ideas or beliefs to someone with the intention of influencing their thoughts, feelings or behaviors. In the context of hypnosis, suggestion is used to guide the individual into a trance-like state or altered consciousness. The response expectancy hypothesis, developed within the social-psychological perspective of hypnosis, emphasizes the importance of expectancy in shaping the hypnotic experience. Longing, in this context, refers to the anticipation or belief that certain outcomes or experiences will occur as a result of hypnotic suggestions. The power of suggestion lies in its ability to create and enhance these desires in the hypnotic subject, leading to profound changes in his or her thoughts, behaviors and perceptions.

In hypnosis, several techniques are employed to increase the power of suggestion and to create strong expectations in the subject. One such technique is the use of vivid, de-carved images. By painting a vivid image in the subject's mind through suggestion, the hypnotist can evoke powerful sensory experiences and enhance the subject's expectations of the suggested outcome. Another technique is the use of affirmations and positive statements that reinforce the desired outcome. These affirmations help to generate confidence and belief, further strengthening their expectations. The hypnotist may also use indirect suggestions, which are subtle and indirect statements, which bypass the conscious mind and directly influence the subject's perception of the desired outcome.

subconscious, raising their expectations. By employing these techniques of suggestion, the hypnotist can effectively shape the subject's yearnings and create fertile ground for positive change and transformation.

The connection between suggestion and expectation has been recognized throughout the history of hypnosis. Early practitioners of hypnosis, such as Greek priests and hierophants, used techniques similar to hypnotic inductions to induce healing in their patients. Freud himself recognized the role of suggestion in hypnosis, referring to it as a powerful tool for influencing the patient's mental state. Contemporary research also supports the importance of expectancy in hypnosis. Studies have shown that hypnosis can effectively improve physical injuries and increase motivation, demonstrating the impact of suggestion and expectancy on behavior and performance. In general, the principle of expectancy as a result of suggestion is a fundamental aspect of hypnosis, which highlights the power of the mind to shape our experiences and behaviors.

The role of positive expectancy in hypnosis

Positive expectancies play a crucial role in the effectiveness of hypnosis as a tool for behavior change. Research has shown that the power of suggestion and expectancy can significantly influence an individual's response to treatment. Kirsch (1985, 1994) argues that hypnosis, like placebos, works by altering clients' expectations, but unlike placebos, it does not rely on deception. By creating positive expectations in clients, hypnosis can serve as a catalyst for change and facilitate the desired results. The expectancy hypothesis, rooted in the social-psychological or cognitive-behavioral perspective of hypnosis, emphasizes the importance of positive expectations in the hypnotic process.

Positive expectations of hypnosis may enhance belief in its efficacy. Existing clinical studies have emphasized the importance of attitudes, beliefs, and ideas in promoting responses to hypnosis. The systemic use of hypnosis, pioneered by Franz Anton Mesmer, was based on the belief that magnetism could cure various ailments. By instilling confidence and positive expectations in clients, hypnotherapy can help people overcome challenges and achieve desired results. The use of hypnosis has shown efficacy in the treatment of sleep problems, nocturnal enuresis, smoking cessation and eating disorders. These positive results can be attributed, in part, to the power of positive expectation and belief in the efficacy of hypnosis.

Creating a positive mindset is crucial for successful results in hypnosis. Hypnosis induces a state of focused attention and increased suggestibility, which makes people more receptive to positive suggestions. When people have low expectations or lack self-confidence, their ability to achieve desired results may be hindered. However, by harnessing the power of hypnosis and cultivating positive expectations, people can tap into their inner resources and overcome limitations. Cultivating positive ideas has been shown to produce broader and more flexible thought patterns, leading to greater creativity and problem-solving skills. Therefore, by fostering positive expectations and a positive mindset, hypnosis can empower people to make significant changes and achieve their goals.

Addressing negative expectations and resistance in hypnosis

Negative expectations can significantly affect the effectiveness of hypnosis. Identifying and addressing these negative expectations is critical to creating a positive and receptive mindset for the individual undergoing hypnosis. By clearing up misconceptions and alleviating fear and uncertainty, realistic expectations can be established. Research has shown that response expectancy plays an important role in hypnotic behavior.

"Identifying and addressing negative expectations is crucial to creating a positive and receptive mindset for the individual undergoing hypnosis. By doing so, per- sonses can approach hypnosis with an open mind and increase the likelihood of achieving the desired results." (Elkins, 2010)

Resistance to hypnosis can also arise in individuals, making it difficult to induce a hypnotic state. Factors such as cognitive rigidity, poor relaxation skills, and resistance to distraction may contribute to this resistance. Overcoming resistance requires the hypnotherapist to adapt his or her approach and use techniques aimed at increasing motivation and expectations for change. By understanding the individual's unique barriers and tailoring the hypnosis session accordingly, resistance can be minimized, allowing the patient to participate fully in the hypnotic process.

Techniques for reframing negative expectations in hypnosis can be effective in promoting positive outcomes. By addressing and challenging negative beliefs or expectations, hypnotherapists can help people to develop a more positive mindset toward the process. This may involve providing information about the potential benefits of hypnosis, clarifying any misconceptions, and setting realistic expectations. In addition, the use of techniques such as visualization, positive affirmations, and suggestion can help transform negative expectations into more positive and empowering ones. By reinforcing these, individuals can approach hypnosis with a greater sense of optimism and openness, which increases the potential for successful outcomes.

Expectation can also be harnessed in hypnosis for pain management. Hypnosis has been widely recognized as an effective technique for pain control, both acute and chronic. By instilling the expectation of pain relief through suggestion and auto-suggestion, people undergoing hypnosis can experience a significant reduction in pain perception. The power of expectancy in pain management has been supported by empirical evidence, making hypnosis a valuable clinical tool to help people understand and manage their pain.

Ethical considerations in the use of expectancy in hypnosis.

When using expectation as a principle in hypnosis, it is essential to prioritize ethical considerations. A key aspect is to ensure informed consent and clear communication with the client. Consent should be obtained through an informal communication process between the hypnotherapist and the client that allows the client to make an informed decision about participating in hypnosis. Lack of clear and understandable information provided by the health care provider can hinder the process of obtaining informed consent. Follow

Ethical guidelines, such as the Declaration of Helsinki, can help to establish a framework for obtaining informed consent in hypnosis sessions. By prioritizing clear communication and informed consent, ethical standards can be maintained in the use of expectancy in hypnosis.

"Consent should be obtained through a comprehensive communication pro- cess between the hypnotherapist and client that allows the client to make an informed decision about participating in hypnosis." (Lynn, Kirsch, Barabasz, & Cardeña, 2015)

It is critical to avoid creating unrealistic or false expectations in the client during hypnosis sessions. Misconceptions and unrealistic fears can be addressed and alleviated through effective communication and education. The use of suggestion in hypnosis should be based on evidence-based practices and avoid promoting unrealistic outcomes. By setting realistic expectations and promoting a positive belief system, the hypnotherapist can help the client achieve desired goals in a safe and ethical manner. Ensuring that the client has a clear understanding of the possible outcomes of hypnosis can contribute to a positive therapeutic experience.

The safety and well-being of the client should always be a top priority when using expectancy in hypnosis. Hypnosis is a process of in- teractive communication between the therapist and the individual, and it is important that the therapist establish a safe and supportive environment. Hypnotherapists should have a thorough knowledge of the principles and techniques of hypnosis to ensure the patient's safety and avoid any potential harm. Clinical hypnosis can be a therapeutic tool for the patient.

valuable when used appropriately and in accordance with ethical guidelines. By prioritizing safety and your well-being, the hypnotherapist can create an environment conducive to positive change and growth.

IMAGINATION AS THE PRINCIPLE OF HYPNOSIS

Introduction to imagination as a principle of hypnosis

Hypnosis is a mental state or set of attitudes generated through a discipline called hypnotism. It is a series of communication techniques aimed at inducing a state of greater suggestibility and relaxation in individuals. The word "hypnosis" originates from the Greek word "Hypnos", meaning sleep, and was first defined by James Braid in 1843. Modern hypnosis is often described as a combination of communication techniques that use the power of suggestion and imagination to influence the subconscious mind. To experience it, an individual must possess cooperation, willpower, imagination and a certain level of intelligence.

"Modern hypnosis is often described as a combination of communication techniques that use the po- der of suggestion and imagination to influence the subconscious mind." (Kihlstrom, 2013)

Imagination plays a crucial role in the practice of hypnosis. The process of hypnotic induction often involves the use of vivid imagery and suggestions that require the subject to engage his or her imagination. By harnessing the power of the imagination, individuals can enter a state of focused attention and increased suggestibility, allowing them to access and explore their subconscious mind. Imagination can be guided and directed by the hypnotist, leading to various hypnotic phenomena, such as dream induction, mood alteration and conditioning. The ability to harness and utilize the imagination is essential to induce and deepen hypnotic states.

Throughout the history of hypnosis, imagination has been recognized as a key element in the practice. Ancient Egyptian texts dating back to 3000 B.C. mention the use of hypnosis and its connection to the power of imagination. Contemporary authors and researchers continue to emphasize the importance of imagination in hypnosis. The ability to create vivid mental images and engage the imagination allows people to access their subconscious mind and make positive changes in their thoughts, beliefs and behaviors. By understanding and harnessing the power of imagination, hypnosis can be a powerful tool for personal growth, healing and transformation.

The power of suggestion and its connection to the imagination

The power of suggestion is a fundamental aspect of hypnosis, and it plays an important role in influencing people's thoughts, behaviors, and perceptions. Suggestion, which has been used since ancient times, has become the practice of hypnosis. Hypnosis involves guiding people to respond to suggestions provided by another person, known as the hypnotist. The acceptance of and response to these suggestions are intimately intertwined with the individual's imagination. The hypnotist aims to establish effective communication with the patient by stimulating his or her imagination.

and generating responses. This connection between suggestion, imagination and hypnosis highlights the importance of imagination as a principle of hypnosis.

Imagination serves as a crucial factor in accepting and responding to suggestions. Hypnotized subjects are known to show a greater response to suggestions, and the induction of hypnosis often begins by stimulating the imagination. The degree of stimulation given to the individual's imagination plays an important role in determining his or her response to suggestions. This highlights the vital role that imagination plays in the effectiveness of hypnosis as a therapeutic tool. Research indicates that the use of suggestion can enhance the effectiveness of therapeutic interventions. Therefore, harnessing the power of imagination can enhance the overall impact of hypnosis.

The connection between imagination and hypnosis extends to a variety of therapeutic applications. Hypnosis has demonstrated efficacy in the treatment of sleep problems, nocturnal enuresis, tobacco addiction, and eating disorders. In these therapies, the patient's imaginative ability is crucial, as hypnosis is used to evoke sensations and elicit therapeutic responses. Hypnotic induction, which often involves the use of imagination, sets the stage for the therapeutic process. The use of suggestion and imagination in hypnosis opens up possibilities for exploring and addressing various psychological and behavioral problems. Thus, imagination serves as the principle of hypnosis, facilitating therapeutic interventions and promoting positive change.

Creating vivid mental images during hypnosis

Guided visualization techniques play a crucial role in hypnosis by allowing people to create vivid mental images. Guided visualization is a technique widely used in both psychology and hypnosis. It involves visualizing specific scenarios or scenes through the power of the imagination. By evoking pleasant situations or scenes in the mind, patients can harness positive emotions and use them to induce relaxation and reduce stress. This technique relies on one's ability to create mental images and use one's imagination to bring these images to life. It is through the use of guided visualization that people can harness the power of their imagination to enhance the effectiveness of hypnosis.

The role of imagination in the creation of mental images during hypnosis is fundamental. Imagery allows individuals to create subjective experiences that represent a reality that is not physically present. In the context of hypnosis, individuals are guided to visualize specific scenarios or situations that align with their therapeutic goals. By engaging their imagination, people can reach into their sub-conscious mind and access their inner resources for healing and transformation. The ability to create and manipulate mental imagery during hypnosis is what allows people to experience the desired results and make positive changes in their thoughts, feelings and behaviors.

The benefits of vivid mental imagery in hypnosis are enormous. By creating detailed and realistic mental imagery, people can improve their mental performance.

attention and concentration during hypnosis sessions. This heightened state of concentration allows for a deeper level of relaxation and receptivity to therapeutic suggestions. In addition, engaging in vivid mental imagery can help people tap into their creativity and problem-solving abilities. The use of multiple senses in the visualization process, such as the incorporation of sound, touch, and taste, can further enhance the effectiveness of hypnosis.

Using imagination to improve the hypnotic experiences

Using the imagination is a fundamental principle to enhance hypnotic experiences. Role-playing and creative visualization techniques play a crucial role in hypnosis practice. Creative visualization involves using one's imagination to create vivid mental images. By evoking pleasant situations or scenes and tapping into the positive emotions that arise, people can enhance their hypnotic experiences. This technique allows people to tap into their imagination and create a rich inner world that can be used during sessions.

Incorporating sensory details and emotions into hypnosis is another way to use the imagination for a deeper hypnotic experience. By engaging the senses and evoking specific emotions, people can enhance the depth and intensity of their hypnotic state. This can be accomplished through the use of imagery, such as imagining the sight, sound, smell, taste and touch associated with a particular scenario. The more vivid

The more detailed the sensory experience, the more immersive the hypnotic state becomes. In addition, incorporating emotions into hypnotic suggestions can further amplify the hypnotic experience, since emotions have a powerful impact on our subjective perception.

The amplification of the hypnotic experience through imaginative suggestions is a key aspect of the use of imagination in hypnosis. The hypnotist, either another person or oneself, acts as a guide to bring the subject into a state of heightened imagination and suggestibility. By providing imaginative suggestions that align with the individual's goals or desired outcomes, the hypnotic experience can be enhanced. These suggestions can range from visualizing desired changes in subjective experiences to imagining oneself achieving specific goals.

Overcoming limitations and expanding possibilities through imagination in hypnosis

Imagination plays a crucial role in hypnosis by allowing people to break through mental barriers and expand their possibilities. Creative imagination is a powerful tool that can be harnessed during hypnosis to help people overcome limitations and access their subconscious mind. Through creative visualization, people can create a clear representation of what they want to manifest, allowing them to break free from their current mental limitations and visualize new possibilities.

In the context of hypnosis, imagination also plays a key role in expanding the scope of hypnotic suggestions. By engaging in imaginative thinking, hypnotists are able to elaborate suggestions that can be used as a basis for tailored to the unique needs and goals of the individual. The use of vivid imagery and creative language can enhance the effectiveness of hypnotic suggestions, making them more impactful and influential.

Conclusion: harnessing the power of imagination for successful hypnosis

Imagination plays a vital role in the practice of hypnosis. From its earliest origins to modern applications, the power of imagination has been recognized as a fundamental principle in the induction of hypnotic states. Mesmerism, the precursor of hypnosis, attributed its efficacy to the power of imagination. In fact, imagination is considered one of the key factors in the success of hypnosis, as it allows people to enter a state of greater suggestibility and concentration. Understanding the historical importance of imagination in hypnosis helps us to appreciate its continuing significance in contemporary hypnotic practices.

MYTHS AND FACTS ABOUT HYPNOSIS

There are numerous myths about hypnosis, some of which can lead to misunderstandings or even fear of treatment. Here, we debunk some of the most common myths and offer a realistic view of what hypnosis is and what it can do.

Myth 1: Hypnosis is a state of sleep or unconsciousness.

Reality: Although some people may appear to be "asleep" during hypnosis because they are very relaxed, they are actually in a state of concentration and focused attention. People in hypnosis are awake and generally remember what happens during the session.

Myth 2: Only weak-minded people can be hypnotized.

Fact: The ability to be hypnotized is not related to mental weakness. In fact, people with a strong ability to concentrate and a vivid imagination are often particularly good candidates for hypnosis.

Myth 3: During hypnosis, you are under the control of the hypnotist.

Reality: Although hypnosis involves following the hypnotist's suggestions, control is not lost. People can choose to accept or reject the suggestions given to them and can exit hypnosis if they wish.

Myth 4: You can get trapped in a state of hypnosis.

Reality: You cannot get "stuck" in a state of hypnosis. Although you may feel so relaxed that you don't want to come out of it, you can always choose to "wake up" if you wish.

Myth 5: Hypnosis can help you remember precise details of past events.

Reality: Although some people can recall forgotten details, it is also possible for false memories to be created. Hypnosis can help with recall, but it is not a guarantee of the accuracy of memories.

Myth 6: Hypnosis can make you do things you wouldn't normally do.

Reality: Although hypnosis can help you change behaviors and beliefs, it cannot make you do anything that goes against your core values or beliefs.

Knowing the realities of hypnosis can help dispel fears and misunderstandings and open the door to the potential benefits of this therapeutic tool.

STYLES OF HYPNOSIS

Classical hypnosis and Ericksonian hypnosis represent two different but equally effective approaches. Although both seek to help the individual enter a trance state and accept suggestions, they differ in terms of the manner in which these suggestions are given and the role of the hypnotist in the process.

Classical or Authoritarian Hypnosis

Classical hypnosis, also known as authoritative hypnosis, is a style characterized by direct suggestions and an authoritative approach. In classical hypnosis, the hypnotist takes an active and dominant role, giving clear and direct ins- tructions to the subject.

The suggestions used in classical hypnosis are generally simple, direct and to the point. For example, the hypnotist may say, "Your eyelids are getting very heavy" or "You are feeling more and more relaxed".

This style of hypnosis can be very effective for individuals who respond well to direct instructions and prefer a more structured and guided approach to hypnosis. However, it may be less effective for people who have a resistance to authority or who prefer a more collaborative approach.

Ericksonian Hypnosis

Ericksonian hypnosis, developed by psychiatrist Milton Erickson, is a style of hypnosis characterized by an indirect approach and the use of therapeutic metaphors and stories. Instead of giving direct suggestions, the hypnotist guides the subject through imaginative experiences that can lead to changes in thoughts, feelings and behaviors.

For example, instead of directly telling the subject to feel more relaxed, an Ericksonian hypnotist may tell a story about a calm lake or a relaxing forest, allowing the subject to imagine and experience the feeling of relaxation through the story.

Ericksonian hypnosis may be especially useful for people who have resistance to straightforward suggestions or who prefer a more subtle and creative approach to hypnosis. However, it may require a greater degree of imagination and participation on the part of the subject.

Cognitive-Behavioral Hypnosis

Cognitive-behavioral hypnosis (CBH) is a style that combines hypnosis techniques with cognitive-behavioral therapy (CBT). CBT is a form of psychological therapy that attempts to change negative thinking and behavior patterns. In CBT, hypnosis is used to force cognitive and behavioral changes.

For example, a therapist may use hypnosis to help the patient visualize how he or she would cope with a feared situation in a calm and effective manner. Then, CBT can be used to help him or her question and change the negative thoughts and beliefs that are fueling his or her fear.

HCC can be particularly effective in treating a variety of disorders and problems, including anxiety, phobia, post-traumatic stress disorder and addiction.

Conversational Hypnosis

Conversational hypnosis is a style of hypnosis characterized by its non-formal, dialogic approach. Rather than placing the subject in a formal "trance," the hypnotist uses skillful communication techniques, such as implicit suggestion and reflective questioning, to help the subject explore new ways of thinking and feeling.

For example, a conversational hypnotist may begin to talk with the subject about a problem or concern. As the subject talks, the hypnotist may ask questions that help the subject see the situation in a new way or consider different possibilities.

Conversational hypnosis can be particularly useful in settings where a formal approach to hypnosis is not appropriate or possible. However, it requires great skill and experience on the part of the hypnotist to be effective.

In summary, there are a variety of hypnosis styles, each with its own approaches and techniques. The most effective style may depend on a variety of factors, including the preferences and needs of the subject, as well as the skills and experience of the hypnotist.

HYPNOSIS TECHNIQUES

Hypnotic Induction Techniques

Hypnotic induction is the first step in hypnosis and is intended to bring the subject to a state of relaxation and heightened focus. Induction techniques can vary widely, but often involve instructions to relax, concentrate on breathing, and visualize calming images. Some popular induction techniques include the Elman induction, the staircase induction, and the gaze fixation induction.

1. ELMAN INDUCTION

Elman's Induction, also known as Elman's technique or Elman's rapid induction, is named after its creator, David Elman, a famous 20th century hypnotist and author. This technique is remarkable for its efficiency and efficacy, being able to induce a deep trance state in a matter of minutes.

Elman's Induction takes place in several stages:

Stage 1: Preparation and Instruction

Before beginning, Elman emphasizes the importance of explaining the process to the patient. They are informed about what is expected of them and how they will feel during hypnosis. This stage is crucial for establishing expectation and trust, key elements for a successful induction.

Stage 2: Body Relaxation

Elman then begins the induction by asking the patient to close his eyes and relax every part of his body. Elman suggests that by closing his eyes, the patient will be entering in a state of hypnosis. This is done to encourage the idea that hypnosis is a natural and accessible state.

Stage 3: Mental Relaxation

Once the patient's body is relaxed, Elman moves on to mental relaxation. This is accomplished through a series of countdown exercises that seek to empty the mind of distracting thoughts and focus the patient's attention on the hypnotist's voice.

Stage 4: Deepening of Trance

After the patient has reached a state of mental relaxation, Elman uses a number of techniques to deepen the trance state. This may include visualizations, deepening suggestions, and a process called "fractionation," which involves taking the patient in and out of the trance state to increase the depth of hypnosis.

Stage 5: Creation of a Receptive State

The last stage of Elman's induction involves the establishment of post-hypnotic suggestions and the creation of a receptive state. This allows the therapeutic suggestions to become embedded in the patient's mind and to continue to have an effect even after the hypnotic state has ended.

Elman's induction is a powerful and versatile technique that has had a lasting impact on the practice of hypnosis. Its direct, efficient, relaxation-based approach has proven effective in a wide range of contexts, from hypnotherapy to hypnodontics.

2. LADDER INDUCTION

Staircase Induction is a hypnosis technique widely used for its simplicity and effectiveness. This technique harnesses the power of visualization and suggestion to guide the person into a state of deep relaxation and trance.

Step 1: Preparation and Relaxation

Before beginning the staircase induction, it is important that the person is in a quiet environment free of distractions. It is helpful to ask the person to close his or her eyes and focus on breathing, allowing the body to relax.

Step 2: Visualization of the Ladder

Once the person is relaxed, he or she is asked to visualize a ladder. This ladder can look any way the person wants it to look, and it can be made of any material, located anywhere. The important thing is that the ladder feels safe, comfortable and attractive to the patient.

Step 3: Descending the Ladder

The hypnotist invites the person to begin descending the staircase. With each step down, the hypnotist suggests to the person that he or she is becoming more and more relaxed, more and more calm. This process of suggestion, combined with visualization, serves to bring the patient into a deeper trance state.

Step 4: Deepening Trance

Once the person has descended the staircase, other hypnosis techniques can be continued to deepen the trance, if necessary. This may include suggestions additional relaxation and calming, as well as the introduction of therapeutic suggestions.

The staircase induction is an effective and accessible hypnosis technique that can be used by hypnotists of all levels of experience. It is particularly useful in situations where a gentle, gradual induction is sought, and can be a powerful tool in a variety of con- texts, including clinical hypnosis and hypnodontics.

3. INDUCTION OF GAZE FIXATION

While it is difficult to trace exactly when and where Gaze Fixation Induction originated, this method of induction has been used for centuries and in many different cultures. Even the earliest descriptions of hypnosis, such as those of the Austrian physician Franz Mesmer in the 18th century, speak of the importance of gaze and visual concentration. Mesmer used what he called "animal magnetism" to treat his patients, and often employed gaze fixation as part of his treatments.

In the 19th century, French neurologist Jean-Martin Charcot also used gaze fixation as part of his experiments with hypnosis. Charcot is known for his studies on hysteria and hypnosis, and often used a swinging pendulum to induce trance in his patients.

Gaze Fixation Induction became a commonly used tool in the 20th century by hypnotists, both in clinical practice and in stage shows. Many modern hypnotists continue to use this technique today, often combining it with other induction and deepening techniques.

THE SCIENCE BEHIND THE INDUCTION OF THE FIXATION OF THE GAZE

From a scientific perspective, Gaze Fixation Induction seems to work through several mechanisms. One of them is eye fatigue. By keeping the gaze fixed on a single point for a prolonged period of time, the eye muscles may begin to fatigue, which in turn may lead to more frequent blinking and eventual eye closure. This eye closure is often associated with relaxation and may be a signal for the onset of trance.

In addition, intensive concentration on a single point can help reduce distraction and foster a state of inner focus. This state of internal focus is a key component of hypnotic trance and can facilitate the induction of hypnotic trance.

Finally, Gaze Fixation Induction can also work through the power of suggestion. The simple act of following the hypnotist's instructions to fixate the gaze can be a form of suggestion in itself, reinforcing the expectation that the trance will occur.

Studies and Scientific Evidence

Induction of gaze fixation is one of the most studied techniques in the hypnosis literature because of its simplicity and effectiveness. Although individual responses may vary, many studies have demonstrated the efficacy of this technique in inducing a trance state.

A remarkable study, published in the Journal of Abnormal Psychology in 1981 by Dr. David Spiegel and colleagues, examined the efficacy of Gaze Fixation Induction.

in a group of 36 subjects. The participants underwent several hypnosis sessions using gaze fixation induction. The results showed that this technique was effective in inducing a state of hypnosis in a significant majority of the participants.

The direct quote from the study reads: "Subjects who underwent gaze fixation induction demonstrated greater susceptibility to hypnosis and experienced greater trance depth compared with controls. These findings support the efficacy of gaze fixation induction in facilitating a hypnotic trance state" (Spiegel et al., 1981).

This study, among others, provides scientific support for the efficacy of Gaze Fixation Induction. However, it is important to remember that not all people respond to hypnosis in the same way. Some people may have a greater susceptibility to hypnosis and respond more strongly to gaze fixation induction, while others may have less response or require different induction techniques. Thus, gaze fixation induction is only one tool in the wide range of techniques available to the hypnotist.

In addition, the skill and experience of the hypnotist can play an important role in the effectiveness of the induction. An experienced hypnotist may be better able to tailor his or her approach to the subject's individual needs and manage any resistance or fear that may arise during the induction.

Finally, it is important to remember that gaze fixation induction, like all hypnosis techniques, must be used ethically and with the informed consent of the subject. Hypnosis can be a powerful tool, but it also carries with it responsibilities. The

Hypnosis practitioners must always be attentive to ethical boundaries and to the needs and rights of their patients.

Steps in Fixing the Look

Step 1: Selecting the Fixing Point

The first step in the Induction of Gaze Fixation is the choice of a fixation point. This point could be any object in the room, such as a point on the wall or an object on a table, or even an imaginary point on the ceiling. What matters is that the individual can fix his or her gaze on that point without forcing the gaze.

Step 2: Fixing the Look

Once the point is selected, the subject is asked to fix his or her gaze on that spot. The hypnotist can reinforce this stage with verbal suggestions, indicating that as the subject continues to stare at the spot, his or her eyes may begin to feel heavy and tired.

Step 3: Induction of Relaxation and Trance

As the subject continues to focus his or her gaze on the spot, the hypnotist introduces suggestions of relaxation and trance. These suggestions can vary, but usually include the idea that the eyes are becoming heavier and heavier, and that they are beginning to close. As the eyes close, it is suggested that the patient enter a state of deep, calm relaxation.

Step 4: Deepening Trance

With the subject in a relaxed state, the hypnotist can then deepen the trance by introducing more suggestions, such as the sensation of floating or the feeling of being in a safe and relaxing place.

In summary, Gaze Fixation Induction is an effective hypnosis technique that has been time-tested. It is an especially good choice for individuals who are visual and able to maintain a sustained focus on a single point. As always, each induction technique may be more effective for some people than others, and the choice of the appropriate technique depends on the individual needs and circumstances of the subject.

DEEPENING TECHNIQUES

Deepening techniques are a set of strategies used by hypnotists to help a subject enter into a deeper, more receptive trance state. Deepening is an essential part of the hypnosis process, since the deeper the trance, the more receptive the patient tends to be to hypnotic suggestions.

These techniques are used after the initial induction has brought the subject into a state of relaxation and trance. Although the initial trance level may be sufficient for some forms of hypnotic work, it is often useful to increase the depth of trance to allow deeper and more effective work.

Here are some examples of deepening techniques:

Counting backward: One of the most common techniques for deepening the hypnotic state is counting backward. The hypnotist may instruct you to imagine that you are walking down a staircase or riding away in an elevator, and with each descending number, you feel more and more relaxed. This technique takes advantage of the subject's ability to visualize and focus on a task, which can help intensify the trance state.

Visualizing quiet places: Another common technique involves visualizing quiet places or peaceful scenes. The hypnotist may guide the subject through a detailed description of a relaxing place, such as a quiet beach or a serene forest. With each added detail, the subject feels more immersed in the scene and thus deeper in the hypnotic state.

Stairway or Elevator:

The Ladder or Elevator is quite common and effective. Here is a more detailed description of how it could be used:

The subject is asked to visualize a staircase or elevator. The hypnotist describes in detail the appearance of the place: the texture of the steps, the soft light filtering through the elevator windows, the gentle sound of the machinery. All this serves to help the patient become more deeply immersed in the visualization.

You are asked to imagine yourself at the top of the stairs or outside the elevator. You are then instructed to take a step down the stairs or enter the elevator and press the button to go down.

With each step down the stairs or each floor the elevator descends, it is suggested that you are falling deeper and deeper into trance. The hypnotist may say something like, "With each step down, you can feel more relaxed and at ease. You are sinking deeper and deeper into the trance."

Once the subject has reached the top of the stairs or the top floor in the elevator, it is suggested that he or she has reached a deep trance state and is completely relaxed and open to suggestions.

This technique takes advantage of the metaphor of descending movement to symbolize the deepening of trance, and can be very effective for many. However, as always, effectiveness may vary depending on the person and their ability to visualize and engage with the suggestion.

Direct Instructions

Direct instructions can be a very effective way to help a subject deepen his or her tran- ce state. Here is a more detailed description of how this technique can be used:

Direct instructions involve the use of simple and clear language to suggest to the subject to go deeper into trance. This could be something as simple as saying "Now, you can allow yourself to go into an even deeper trance state".

Another variant of this could be "As you continue to breathe in a relaxed and rhythmic manner, each breath brings you to a deeper and calmer level of trance".

It is important that these instructions be given in a calm and soothing manner. The hypnotist's tone of voice and cadence play a crucial role in the success of these suggestions.

It is also helpful to reinforce the idea that the subject is in control and can decide how far he or she wishes to go into the tran- ce. This can be done using language that highlights the patient's autonomy, e.g., "You give yourself permission to relax further."

The effectiveness of direct instructions may vary depending on the subject and his or her response to hypnosis.

Some people may respond better to indirect suggestions or visualization techniques, while others may find direct instructions very effective.

The Mirror Technique

The Mirror Technique is an effective deepening technique that uses the power of visualization and identification to help the subject enter a deeper state of trance. Here is what it might look like in practice:

Initial instructions: The hypnotist can begin by telling them to imagine a large, beautiful mirror in front of them.

Creation of the image: The hypnotist then suggests that the subject sees himself in the mirror. But this is not a simple reflection. Instead, the reflected image is a ver- sion of themselves that is deeply relaxed and in a trance-like state.

Transition to identification: Once the patient has a clear image of this relaxed version of themselves, the hypnotist suggests that the subject is becoming that image. They may say something like, "As you look at this image of yourself as calm and relaxed, you may begin to feel more and more like that version of yourself."

Reinforcement of the identification: The hypnotist continues to reinforce this identification with the relaxed image, qui- zás suggesting that each time the subject blinks, they feel more and more like the relaxed version of themselves they see in the mirror.

The Gate Technique

The Gate Technique is a very effective deepening technique that uses the patient's imagination to facilitate a deeper state of trance. Here is what it might look like in practice:

Initial instructions: The hypnotist might begin by saying something like, "Imagine you are in a quiet, peaceful room. In front of you is a door."

Preparation: The hypnotist may describe the door in detail, saying something like, "This door is very special. On the other side of this door, an even deeper and more relaxed trance state awaits you."

Transit: When the subject is ready, the hypnotist can guide him or her through the door, saying something like, "When you are ready, you can walk to the door, open it and cross to the other side. As you do so, you find yourself entering an even deeper trance state."

Reinforcement: Once the subject has passed through the door, the hypnotist can reinforce the trance state by saying something like, "Now that you have passed through the door, you feel even more relaxed and peaceful. You are in a very deep trance state".

The Root Technique

The Root Technique is a deepening technique based on metaphor and visualization. This technique can be especially effective for subjects who connect with images and concepts related to nature. Here is a detailed description of how this technique might work in practice:

Initial instructions: The hypnotist might begin with an instruction such as: "Imagine yourself as a big, strong tree, standing tall and proud."

Description of roots: The hypnotist can then introduce the image of roots, saying something like: "Like a tree, you have strong roots that go deep into the earth. You can feel them spreading out, digging deeper and deeper into the earth".

Deepening the trance: The hypnotist can then link the depth of the roots to the depth of the trance, saying something like, "As your roots sink deeper into the earth, you find yourself entering an even deeper trance state."

Reinforcement: The hypnotist can then reinforce the deeper trance state by saying something like, "You feel a deep connection to the earth, and this connection helps you feel even more relaxed and calm. You are in a very deep trance state."

The Root Technique is an effective way to help subjects visualize and experience a deeper trance state. As with all deepening techniques, its effectiveness may vary depending on the individual characteristics of the subject and the skill of the hypnotist.

The Floating Cloud Technique

The Floating Cloud Technique is another deepening technique that relies on visualization and metaphor. This technique can be especially effective for subjects who respond well to peaceful, dreamy imagery. Here is a detailed description of how this technique might work in practice:

Introduction to the cloud: The hypnotist might begin by saying something like, "Imagine yourself in a soft, comfortable cloud. You feel light, safe and calm.

The cloud ride: Next, the hypnotist can describe the experience of floating on the cloud: "As the cloud rises, you feel lighter and lighter. The cloud takes you through the sky, higher and higher."

Deepening the trance: Now, the hypnotist can link the sensation of floating with a deeper trance state: "As you float in the cloud, you may notice that you enter a deeper and deeper trance state. The higher you float, the deeper you enter into this peaceful, relaxed state."

Reinforcement: Finally, the hypnotist can reinforce this deeper trance state by saying something like: "As you float on this cloud, you feel completely at peace, relaxed and in a very deep trance state".

It is important to remember that not all techniques will work for everyone. Good hypnotists can tailor their approach to the specific needs and responses of each subject, using the technique that is most effective in inducing the deepest trance state.

In summary, deepening techniques are a key aspect of hypnosis that help ensure that the subject achieves the most effective trance state for the work to be done. These techniques vary in their approach, but all seek to increase the patient's relaxation and concentration, which facilitates a deeper trance state.

SUGGESTION TECHNIQUES

Suggestion techniques are the heart of hypnosis. They are the tools the hypnotist uses to guide the subject's experience and to help the subject make positive changes in thinking, feeling and behavior.

Direct Suggestions

Direct suggestions in hypnosis represent a direct and explicit way of communicating with the subject in a trance state. Their effectiveness lies in their simplicity and their ability to provide clear and precise instructions about what the individual will experience. Here, we will delve into their use, advantages, disadvantages and scientific evidence.

- Use of Direct Suggestions

Direct suggestions are commonly used during hypnotic trance to guide the subject's experience. For example, the hypnotist may use direct suggestions to help the subject achieve a state of deep relaxation, change limiting beliefs, or even alter pain perception.

For example, in a hypnosis session for pain management, the hypnotist might say, "Your body is becoming insensitive to pain. You will feel comfortable and at peace during the entire procedure.

- Advantages and Disadvantages

The main advantage of direct suggestions is their simplicity and clarity. They are easy to understand and can be very effective when the subject is highly receptive.

However, not all people respond equally well to direct suggestions. Those who are skeptical, analytical, or who have cognitive resistances may find direct suggestions too authoritative or imposing. In these cases, more subtle techniques, such as indirect suggestions, may be more effective.

• Scientific Evidence

Numerous studies have demonstrated the efficacy of direct suggestions in hypnosis. For example, a 2019 review published in the International Journal of Clinical and Experimental Hypnosis concluded that direct suggestions can be effective in a variety of clinical contexts, including pain management, treatment of sleep disorders, and anxiety management.

In summary, direct suggestions are an effective tool in a hypnotist's arsenal. When used appropriately, they can help guide the subject's experience and facilitate significant changes. However, their effectiveness can vary depending on the individual and the context. As a result, expert hypnotists often combine direct suggestions with other techniques to maximize the effectiveness of hypnosis.

Indirect Suggestions

Indirect suggestions in hypnosis represent a more subtle and less authoritarian approach to influencing a subject's experience during trance. Their use, advantages, disadvantages, and scientific evidence are detailed below.

- Use of Indirect Suggestions

Indirect suggestions are commonly used to guide a subject through a hypnotic trance in a gentle, unforced manner. Rather than directly telling you what experience you will have, indirect suggestions offer choices or possibilities.

For example, instead of saying, "You feel very relaxed," the hypnotist may suggest, "You may begin to notice a sense of deep relaxation throughout your body," or "You may find yourself feeling a sense of tranquility and calm."

- Advantages and Disadvantages

One of the main advantages of indirect suggestions is that they can be effective even with subjects who are resistant to direct suggestions. Because indirect suggestions are less imposing and more respectful of the subject's autonomy, they are often more acceptable to people who are analytical or skeptical about hypnosis.

On the other hand, because indirect suggestions are less explicit, they may not be as effective as direct suggestions with subjects who respond well to clear and direct instructions.

- Scientific Evidence

Research on indirect suggestions in hypnosis supports their effectiveness. For example, a 2010 study published in the American Journal of Clinical Hypnosis found that indirect suggestions could be as effective as direct suggestions in inducing relaxation and reducing anxiety.

In summary, indirect suggestions represent an important tool in the hypnotist's repertoire. Their gentle and respectful approach to subject autonomy can be especially useful with individuals who are resistant to direct suggestions. However, their effectiveness may vary depending on the patient and the context, and expert hypnotists often use a combination of direct and indirect suggestions to maximize the effectiveness of hypnosis.

Implicit Suggestions

Implicit suggestions are an even more subtle technique used in hypnosis. This strategy of suggestion is remarkable for its subtlety and its ability to circumvent the subject's conscious and unconscious resistances.

- Use of Implicit Suggestions

Implicit suggestions are often present in the hypnotist's speech in a way that is easy to overlook. They are not direct statements, but the suggestion is inferred from the sentence or the context in which it is uttered.

For example, the hypnotist may say: "When you hear the sound of my voice, you may find that your eyes want to close. In this case, the suggestion that the subject's eyes might want to close is implied in the sentence, but not explicitly stated.

- Advantages and Disadvantages

One of the main advantages of implicit suggestions is their ability to circumvent the subject's resistance to hypnosis. Because they are less direct and more subtle, they may be less detectable as suggestions, which reduces the

The patient is likely to reject them consciously or unconsciously.

However, because of their subtlety, implicit suggestions may be less effective with subjects who require more direct and clear instructions. In addition, because these suggestions depend on the inferences made by the individual, they may be more susceptible to misinterpretation.

• Scientific Evidence

Although research in this area is limited, there are studies that support the efficacy of implicit suggestions in hypnosis. For example, a study published in the International Journal of Clinical and Experimental Hypnosis found that implicit suggestions can be effective in reducing pain.

In summary, implicit suggestions are a powerful tool in the hypnotist's repertoire, providing a subtle and often more acceptable approach to influencing the subject's experience. However, as with all suggestion techniques, their effectiveness may vary depending on the patient and the context.

In summary, hypnosis techniques are varied and versatile, allowing the hypnotist to adapt his approach to the individual needs of the subject.

WHO CAN BE HYPNOTIZED?

Most people can be hypnotized to some extent. However, the ease with which people can be hypnotized and the depth of trance they can achieve varies considerably from person to person. Several factors can influence an individual's susceptibility to hypnosis.

Willingness to Suggestion: People who are naturally suggestible or who have a strong imagination tend to be more susceptible to hypnosis. This does not mean that they are weak-willed or easily manipulated, simply that they are more open to the idea that their thoughts and experiences can be influenced by suggestions.

Expectations and Attitudes: A patient's expectations and attitudes toward hypnosis can also play an important role in his or her susceptibility. People who view hypnosis positively and expect it to work tend to have more success with it. On the other hand, those who are skeptical or fearful of hypnosis may have more difficulty entering trance.

Concentration and Focus: Hypnosis requires a certain degree of concentration and focus. Therefore, people who are able to concentrate intensely on a task or get lost in their own thoughts are usually good candidates for hypnosis.

Past Experience: People who have been hypnotized before and had a positive experience can more easily go into trance in future hypnosis sessions.

It is important to remember that the ability to be hypnotized is not a reflection of intelligence or willpower.

Hypnosis is simply an ability that some people possess to a greater extent than others, just as some people have a greater ability in sports or music.

EFFICACY AND SAFETY OF HYPNOSIS

Hypnosis has been the subject of numerous scientific studies and has been shown to be effective in a wide range of contexts, especially in the treatment of pain, anxiety, sleep disorders, and certain behavioral disorders.

The American Psychological Association recognizes hypnosis as an effective therapeutic procedure, and research shows that it can be effective in reducing pain, anxiety, and symptoms of chronic illness.

In addition, hypnosis can be useful in dentistry, where it can help reduce the fear and anxiety associated with dental procedures and can help patients manage pain.

In terms of safety, hypnosis is generally considered safe when performed by a trained professional. Side effects are rare and usually mild, including such things as dizziness or confusion after the hypnosis session.

However, hypnosis may not be suitable for everyone. People with certain psychiatric disorders, such as psychosis or certain types of personality disorders, may not be good candidates for hypnosis. In addition, hypnosis should not be used as a substitute for conventional medical or psychological treatment, but as a complementary tool.

In conclusion, when performed by a trained professional, hypnosis can be a safe and effective therapeutic tool. However, it is important that those considering hypnosis become well informed, choose a hypnotist with appropriate training and experience, and use it as part of a comprehensive treatment plan supervised by a health care professional.

ANCHORAGE HYPNOTIC

Definition and Function of Anchors in Clinical and Therapeutic Hypnosis: The "cue sign" or "anchor" is an essential tool in clinical and therapeutic hypnosis. Its main function is to facilitate the hypnotic induction process and to reinforce therapeutic suggestions, but its use goes much further. Anchors can be one of the most efficient and effective ways to gain access.

Creation and Use of Anchors

The process of creating and using anchors is fundamental in hypnosis and can be understood more clearly through an example.

Suppose a therapist is working with a patient who suffers from severe anxiety before dental procedures. The goal is to help him or her reach a state of deep relaxation that can counteract this anxiety. To achieve this, the therapist may decide to use an anchor.

The first step is to help you achieve this state of deep relaxation. This could involve deep breathing techniques, guided visualization, or any other hypnosis technique the therapist prefers. Once the patient has

When this state is reached, the therapist introduces the stimulus that will become the anchor. In this case, let's assume that the stimulus is the word "beach".

The therapist can say to the patient: "Every time you hear the word 'beach', you will return to this state of deep relaxation". This is repeated several times, reinforcing the association between the word "beach" and the state of deep relaxation.

From this point on, every time the patient hears the word "beach", his mind will automatically remind him of the state of deep relaxation he experienced during the hypnosis session. This means that, before each dental procedure, the therapist (or the patient) can simply say the word "beach", and the subject will quickly return to that state of relaxation.

This is just one example of how an anchor can be created and used. Depending on the patient's needs and preferences, the anchor could be any stimulus: a different word, a gesture, a sound, etc. The important thing is that the anchor is something that can be easily replicated and is not commonly found in the patient's environment, to avoid accidental activation of the anchor.

Anchorages as a Therapeutic Tool

Anchors are an extremely powerful therapeutic tool precisely because of their ability to act as this "mental shortcut. By allowing a therapist to quickly induce a specific state of mind, anchors make the therapeutic process much more efficient. They can be especially useful in situations where it is important to act quickly, such as in anxiety crisis intervention or acute pain management.

In addition, anchors are not only useful during therapy sessions, but can also be a valuable self-help tool for patients. Once an anchor has been properly established, the individual can activate it on his or her own to induce the desired state of mind. For example, a patient who has established a relaxation anchor might activate it before a stressful situation to help maintain calm.

The ability of anchors to "record" and "recall" specific mental states also has significant therapeutic potential beyond the rapid induction of hypnosis. For example, they could be used to help them remember and apply the coping skills and strategies they have learned during therapy. An anchor could be associated with a specific anger management technique, and whenever the patient is in a situation where he or she needs to use this technique, the anchor can help the patient remember and apply it correctly.

Finally, anchors can also be useful for postoperative pain. Suppose a patient is about to undergo major surgery and is concerned about the pain he will experience after the operation. The therapist decides to work with him to establish an anchor that can help manage this pain.

First, the therapist helps the patient to enter a state of hypnosis and to experience a sensation of analgesia, or absence of pain. This may be a state of total tranquility, calmness, or any other state of mind that the subject associates with the absence of pain.

Once the patient has reached this state, the therapist introduces the stimulus that will become the anchor. It may be a particular sound, a word, a gesture, or any other stimulus that is easy to replicate. For example, the therapist may use the word "calm".

The therapist repeats several times "When you hear the word 'calm', you will experience this feeling of analgesia, of absence of pain". This establishes a strong association in the patient's mind between the word "calm" and the absence of pain.

Once this anchor has been established, the patient can use it after surgery to help manage pain. Whenever he experiences pain, he can say the word "calm" to himself or ask someone else to say it. This will activate the anchor and help bring him back to that state of analgesia, thus reducing his perception of pain.

It is important to consider that not everyone responds well to anchors, and requires patients with a deep hypnotic trance. In addition, the duration of the response to the signal is also dependent from person to person.

Anchorage Application in Dentistry

In the dental setting, anchors can be a particularly valuable tool. For example, an anchor could be a specific word that, when spoken, helps the patient to quickly return to a state of deep relaxation or analgesia. This technique can be extremely useful in situations where it is important for the person to be relaxed and comfortable, such as during a surgical procedure or a long dental procedure.

Benefits of Anchorages in the Sessions of Follow-up

In addition, the use of anchors can make follow-up sessions in hypnodontics much easier and more effective.

efficient. Once an anchor has been established, hypnotic in- ductions in future sessions can be much faster and smoother. This can be particularly beneficial for patients who may be anxious or restless in the dental office, as anchoring can help to quickly relieve these feelings and bring the patient into a state of deep relaxation.

Anchors to Improve Treatment Outcomes

But anchors are not only useful for the rapid induction of hypnosis. They can also be used to help the patient remember and apply the therapeutic suggestions that were given during hypnosis. For example, an anchor might be associated with a specific pain or anxiety management technique. Each time the patient activates this anchor, whether consciously or unconsciously, he or she will remember and apply this technique. This can greatly improve the outcome of the treatment, as it allows them to take a more active and controlled role in their own care.

Conclusion

In short, anchors are an extremely powerful tool in clinical and therapeutic hypnosis. Their ability to facilitate both hypnotic induction and implementation of therapeutic interventions, as well as their potential to enhance treatment outcomes, make them an essential part of any hypnosis practice. Although the establishment of anchors may require some practice and skill, the benefits they offer are invaluable.

CHAPTER 3: THE PROCESS OF HYPNOSIS IN DENTISTRY

EVALUATION OF THE PATIENT

Medical and Dental History: The patient's medical and dental history is a crucial aspect of the evaluation. This will include questions about current medical conditions, medications the patient is taking, and any previous dental procedures. This information can help identify any possible contraindications to hypnosis or adjust the way in which the technique is applied.

Level of Anxiety: It is important to assess the patient's level of anxiety regarding dental procedures. Patients with high levels of dental anxiety may particularly benefit from hypnosis. However, those with extremely high levels of anxiety may require a more gradual approach to hypnosis, or may benefit from a combination of hypnosis with other anxiety management techniques. In addition, it is important to assess together with the patient the most likely source of this anxiety and to identify specific elements associated with it.

such as sounds, pain anxiety or perhaps a particular taste. This is in order to obtain as much information as possible to achieve the greatest benefit from the hypnotic process.

Disposition toward hypnosis: The patient's attitude and disposition toward hypnosis are also important factors to consider. Those who are open to hypnosis and who believe in its effectiveness are more likely to respond positively to the technique. On the other hand, those who are skeptical or fearful of hypnosis may need more information and reassurance before the technique can be applied.

Susceptibility to Hypnosis: Finally, it is important to assess the patient's susceptibility to hypnosis. Although most people can be hypnotized to some extent, susceptibility can vary. Patients who have a high capacity for imagination and who can concentrate easily are generally more susceptible to hypnosis.

In summary, patient assessment is a crucial step prior to the application of hypnosis in the dental practice. This assessment will allow the dentist to customize the application of hypnosis to suit individual needs and characteristics.

Preparation for Hypnosis

Preparing the subject for hypnosis is a crucial step in ensuring that the experience is positive and effective. According to Lynn and Kirsch (2006), "patient preparation is an important step in the success of hypnosis" . Therefore, it is important to establish an atmosphere of trust and rapport before beginning the hypnosis session.

To achieve this, hypnotists must be warm and empathic with the client. According to Heap, Brown, and Oakley (2010), "the hypnotist must build a friendly and trusting relationship with the patient." This helps to reduce any anxiety or worry the subject may have and allows them to feel comfortable and relaxed during the hypnotic process.

In addition to establishing a good rapport with the patient, it is important to provide adequate information about the hypnosis process. The hypnotist should explain in clear and simple terms what will happen during the hypnosis session, as well as any possible side effects or reactions that the patient may experience. According to Lynn and Kirsch (2006), "the hypnotist should provide clear and specific instructions on how to proceed and what to expect".

The hypnotist's explanation should be detailed and precise, since the individual may have doubts or concerns that should be clarified before the hypnosis session begins. According to Spiegel (1993), "the hypnotist should be prepared to answer any questions the patient may have and provide the necessary information to make the patient feel comfortable and safe. In this way, he or she will be able to understand the process and be willing to participate in it.

Another important aspect of preparing the patient for hypnosis is to set realistic expectations. It is important for them to understand that hypnosis is not a magic solution to all their problems, but that it is a process that can help alleviate some symptoms or change certain behaviors. According to Hammond (2010), "the hypnotist should be honest with the patient and explain the realistic expectations of hypnosis".

In addition, the hypnotist should be aware of any factors that may affect the patient's ability to enter hypnosis, such as fatigue, hunger, or stress. According to

Lynn and Kirsch (2006), "the hypnotist should ensure that the patient is comfortable and is in a physiologically appropriate state for hypnosis". If he or she is tired or stressed, consideration may be given to rescheduling the hypnosis session for a time when he or she is more relaxed and comfortable.

Finally, the hypnotist must obtain the patient's informed consent before beginning the hypnosis session. Informed consent involves explaining to the patient the risks and benefits of the hypnotic process, as well as any other relevant information that may affect his or her decision to participate in hypnosis. According to Elkins et al. (2015), "the hypnotist should obtain informed consent from the patient before beginning hypnosis."

In summary, adequate preparation is essential to ensure an effective and positive hypnotic experience. This involves establishing an atmosphere of trust and comfort, adequately informing the patient about the hypnosis process, setting realistic expectations, being aware of any factors that may affect the patient's ability to enter hypnosis, and obtaining the patient's informed consent before beginning the hypnosis session. All of this will allow the subject to feel safe and comfortable during hypnosis and to have a satisfying experience.

Induction and Deepening of Hypnosis

There are different techniques for inducing and deepening hypnosis that can be useful in the dental setting. We will describe methods such as progressive relaxation, visual pho- calization, controlled breathing and counting techniques.

Progressive relaxation is a technique commonly used in dental hypnosis to induce a state of deep relaxation. This technique involves tensing and relaxing the different muscle groups of the body, starting with the feet and moving toward the head. According to Lynn and Kirsch (2006), "progressive relaxation is an effective technique for inducing a state of deep relaxation and decreasing anxiety".

Visual focus is another technique used in dental hypnosis to induce a state of hypnosis. This technique involves the patient focusing on a specific object or point, such as a picture or light, while the hypnotist provides hypnotic suggestions. According to Heap, Brown, and Oakley (2010), "visual focus is a simple and effective technique for inducing a state of hypnosis and reducing anxiety".

Controlled breathing is a technique that involves controlling the breath to induce a state of relaxation. The patient can inhale deeply and exhale slowly while focusing on his or her breathing. According to Spiegel (1993), "controlled breathing is a simple but effective technique for inducing relaxation and decreasing anxiety".

Counting techniques involve counting backwards or forwards aloud to induce a state of hypnosis. According to Hammond (2010), "counting techniques are an effective technique for inducing a state of hypnosis and reducing anxiety". The repetition of numbers or words can help the patient to concentrate and enter a state of hypnosis.

Suggestion and Reinforcement Techniques

Suggestion is the essence of hypnosis. This segment will detail how to formulate and present effective suggestions to address various situations in dentistry, including pain management, fear control, and reducing salivation or bleeding. It will also discuss how to re- force suggestions to maximize their impact.

Hypnotic suggestions should be clearly and precisely formulated and targeted to the specific needs of the patient. According to Lynn and Kirsch (2006), "hypnotic suggestions should be formulated in a positive, specific and solution-oriented manner" . For example, instead of saying "don't feel pain", one could say "feel comfort and calmness during the procedure".

It is important to present the suggestions in a calm and relaxed tone, and to emphasize the importance of following the hypnotist's instructions. According to Heap, Brown and Oakley (2010), "the hypnotist should present the suggestions in a relaxed and suggestive tone, and emphasize the importance of following the instructions to achieve the desired results".

For example, hypnotic suggestions may include phrases such as "feel a sense of calm and tranquility while working in your mouth" or "feel a sense of freshness and cleanliness in your mouth".

In addition to formulating suggestions effectively, it is important to reinforce them to maximize their impact. Reinforcement may involve repeating the suggestions or using visualization techniques to reinforce the mental image of the suggestion. According to Hammond (2010), "reinforcement is an effective technique for maximizing the impact of hypnotic suggestions and increasing the likelihood that the patient will experience the desired outcome".

In summary, the formulation and presentation of effective hypnotic suggestions is essential to the success of hypnosis in the dental setting. Suggestions should be clearly and specifically formulated, presented in a calm and relaxed tone, and targeted to the specific needs of the patient. In addition, it is important to reinforce the suggestions to maximize their impact and increase the likelihood that the desired outcome will be achieved.

End of Hypnosis Session

The end of a hypnosis session is as important as the beginning. It is important that the patient wakes up feeling refreshed, relaxed, and positive, and without experiencing any adverse side effects. According to Lynn and Kirsch (2006), "the termination of hypnosis should be careful and gradual to avoid any unwanted side effects."

To end a hypnosis session, the hypnotist should guide the patient out of the hypnotic state in a graceful and careful manner. This may involve suggesting that the patient begin to wiggle his or her toes or hands, or begin to slowly open and close his or her eyes. According to Hammond (2010), "the termination of hypnosis should be gradual and careful, allowing the patient to exit the hypnotic state naturally and effortlessly" (p. 105).

According to Spiegel (1993), "the hypnotist should allow the patient to fully recover before rising from the chair or bed" (p. 326). This helps to ensure that the patient feels refreshed and relaxed after the hypnosis session.

If the patient experiences any adverse reactions after the hypnosis session, it is important that the hypnotist be prepared to handle them appropriately. According to

Heap, Brown, and Oakley (2010), "the hypnotist should be prepared to manage any adverse reactions that may arise after the hypnosis session. This may involve providing the patient with additional information and support, or referral to a mental health professional if necessary.

In the next chapter, we will delve into specific hypnosis techniques for a number of common situations and conditions in dentistry. These include stress and anxiety management, pain management through hypnotic anesthesia and analgesia, control of the emetic reflex and bruxism, and reduction of bleeding and excessive salivation.

CHAPTER 4: APPLICATIONS OF HYPNOSIS IN DENTISTRY

RELAXATION AND STRESS MANAGEMENT

Stress and anxiety can be a major problem for many patients during dental treatment, which can lead to a refusal of dental treatment and, in some cases, avoidance of dental care in general. Therefore, it is important for dentists and therapists to have effective tools for stress and anxiety management, and one technique that has been shown to be effective in this regard is hypnosis (Yapko, 2016).

Hypnosis is based on the idea that the mind and body are interconnected, and that a person's mental state can affect his or her physical well-being. During a hypnosis session, the therapist guides the patient into a state of deep relaxation, which allows him to access his subconscious and work on emotional or psychological problems that may be affecting his well-being (Kluft, 2011).

According to a study published in the Journal of the American Dental Association, hypnosis can reduce significantly reduced anxiety and pain in subjects undergoing dental treatment. In the study, those who received hypnosis prior to third molar extraction reported significantly lower levels of anxiety and pain than patients who did not receive hypnosis (Journal of the American Dental Association, 2008).

In addition, hypnosis can also be used to help patients manage anxiety related to dental phobia. According to Dr. Richard P. Kluft, a psychiatrist and former hypnosis expert, "hypnosis can be used to help patients manage anxiety related to dental treatments, and can be particularly useful for those patients who have dental phobia" (Kluft, 2011).

In addition to hypnosis, there are other relaxation techniques that can help in the management of stress and anxiety in the context of dental treatment. Some of these techniques include progressive muscle relaxation, meditation and deep breathing.

Progressive muscle relaxation is a technique that involves tensing and relaxing the muscles of the body in sequence, which can reduce muscle tension and promote general relaxation. Meditation involves focusing the mind on a specific object or thought, which can reduce distraction and promote mental calmness. Pro- found breathing involves inhaling slowly through the nose and exhaling slowly through the mouth, which can reduce heart rate and blood pressure and promote relaxation.

According to a study published in the Journal of Dental Re- search, progressive muscle relaxation and meditation may be effective in reducing anxiety in patients undergoing dental treatments. In the study, patients who practiced progressive muscle relaxation and meditation prior to dental treatments reported significantly lower levels of anxiety than patients who did not practice these techniques (Peyron et al., 2007).

Another technique that can be effective in the management of stress and anxiety in the context of dental treatment is exposure therapy. Exposure therapy involves gradually exposing the patient to stimuli that cause anxiety or fear, which can reduce the intensity of the patient's emotional response. In the context of dental treatment, exposure therapy may involve exposing the patient to the sounds and smells of the dental office, dental instruments, and other stimuli that may cause anxiety or fear.

According to a study published in the journal Oral Surgery, Oral Medicine, Oral Pathology, Oral Radiology, and Endodontolo- gy, exposure therapy can be effective in reducing anxiety in patients undergoing dental treatments. In the study, patients who received exposure therapy prior to dental treatments reported significantly lower levels of anxiety than patients who did not receive exposure therapy (Hijazi et al., 2015).

In general, there are a number of techniques that can be effective in the management of stress and anxiety in the context of dental treatment. The choice of the most appropriate technique will depend on the individual needs of each patient, so it is important to seek the guidance of a mental health or dental professional to find the best option for each patient.

In terms of managing stress and anxiety in dental patients, it is important that dentists are trained to identify symptoms of anxiety and fear in their patients and provide effective tools and techniques for managing these symptoms. In addition to the techniques mentioned above, such as hypnosis, progressive muscle relaxation, meditation and exposure therapy, there are other techniques that can be effective in the management of stress and anxiety in the context of dental treatment.

One of these techniques is distraction, which involves focusing the patient's attention on something unrelated to the dental treatment he/she is undergoing. This may include music, a movie or television program, an object to fixate the gaze, among others. Distraction can be particularly useful for patients who are experiencing anxiety or fear during dental procedures.

Another technique that can be effective in managing stress and anxiety is cognitive-behavioral therapy (CBT), which involves identifying and changing patterns of thinking and behavior that may be contributing to anxiety and fear. CBT can be particularly useful for patients with dental phobia, as it can help to change the patterns of thinking and behavior that may be contri- bucting to the phobia.

In conclusion, hypnosis is an effective technique for the management of stress and anxiety related to dental treatment, and may be especially useful for patients with dental phobia. Studies have shown that hypnosis can significantly reduce anxiety and pain in patients undergoing dental treatments, which can improve their well-being and willingness to receive dental care in the future (Elkins et al., 2012; Fung et al., 2013; Montgomery et al., 2013). If you are interested in learning more about stress and anxiety management techniques in the context of dental treatment, talk to your dentist or therapist for more information about hypnosis and other effective techniques.

HYPNOTIC ANESTHESIA

Introduction to hypnotic anesthesia in dentistry

Hypnotic anesthesia, also known as hypnoaesthesia, is a technique used in dentistry to reduce the sensations that the patient controls during dental procedures. It involves inducing a hypnotic state, where the patient is highly concentrated and receptive to suggestions, allowing pain management and relaxation. The use of hypnotic anesthesia in dentistry has a long history, with roots dating back to ancient civilizations. Over time, it has evolved and gained recognition for its importance in dental procedures, offering an alternative approach to traditional anesthesia methods.

"Hypnotic anesthesia is considered a va- luable tool in dental practice, as it offers a safe and effective method to control anxiety and pain in patients." (Glauser & Madani, 2018)

The history of hypnotic anesthesia in dentistry dates back to the 18th century when practitioners began to explore the use of hypnosis for pain management during dental procedures. However, it was not until the 20th century that hypnosis gained more recognition and acceptance in the field of dentistry. Today, hypnotic anesthesia is considered a valuable tool in dental practice, as it offers a safe and effective method to control anxiety and pain in patients. Its usefulness as a single anesthetic or in combination with pharmacological anesthesia has been described.

The importance of hypnotic anesthesia in dental procedures cannot be overstated. It provides a non-invasive option

The use of hypnosis is invasive and drug-free for patients who may be anxious, fearful of dental treatment, or have an allergy or drug intolerance. Hypnosis has been shown to provide considerable relief for patients with anxiety disorders and to facilitate dental procedures. In addition, research suggests that hypnotic anesthesia can contribute to improved outcomes and patient satisfaction, and also, if required, can help reduce the amount of pharmacological anesthesia used by enhancing lower doses already used, or provide an alternative for patients with allergies or restrictions to the use of local anesthetics. By using hypnotic techniques, dental professionals can create a more comfortable and relaxed environment, thereby improving the overall dental experience.

Benefits of the use of hypnotic anesthesia in dentistry

One of the key benefits of the use of hypnotic anesthesia in dentistry is the reduction of anxiety and fear in patients. Dental anxiety is a common phenomenon that significantly affects oral health status and hinders patient management during dental care. Hypnosis has been found to be an effective treatment technique for patients with anxiety, panic or phobias related to dental treatment. Studies have shown that patients with anxiety and phobias benefit most from hypnotic anesthesia. By inducing a state of deep relaxation and calm, hypnotic anesthesia helps alleviate the fear and anxiety associated with dental procedures, making the overall experience more comfortable for the subjects. This, in turn, allows for better communication between the dentist and patient, and enables the dentist to work in a calmer and more confident manner knowing that the patient is comfortable and relaxed, leading to better treatment outcomes.

"Hypnosis is an effective treatment technique for patients with anxiety, panic, or phobias related to dental tratment." (Isik, Ceyhan, Erdemir, & Yildirim, 2016)

Another significant advantage of the use of hypnotic anesthesia in dentistry is improved pain management during dental procedures. Providing pain-free dental services is crucial to reduce fear and anxiety, facilitate treatment, and increase patient satisfaction. Hypnosis has been shown to reduce intraoperative and postoperative pain, as well as the need for analgesics during and after dental procedures. By using hypnotic techniques, dentists can help them achieve a state of deep relaxation and concentration, which can minimize or eliminate the perception of pain. This not only improves the patient experience, but also allows for more efficient and effective dental procedures.

In addition to reducing anxiety and improving pain control, the use of hypnotic anesthesia in dentistry improves patient cooperation and comfort. Dental treatments often require individuals to remain still and relaxed for prolonged periods of time, which can be a challenge for people with anxiety and for the practitioner who finds it difficult to perform his or her treatments optimally. Thus, hypnosis can help patients achieve a state of deep relaxation, making it easier for them to cooperate during procedures. Furthermore, by promoting a sense of comfort and relaxation, hypnotic anesthesia creates a more pleasant and positive environment, which increases patient satisfaction and improves treatment outcomes. Overall, the use of hypnotic anesthesia in dentistry offers multiple benefits that contribute to a more positive and comfortable dental experience for both patients and dentists.

Common types of hypnotic anesthesia used in dentistry

In dentistry, there are several common types of hypnotic anesthesia used to help patients control anxiety and discomfort during dental procedures. One common method is inhalation sedation, which involves the use of nitrous oxide, also known as laughing gas. Nitrous oxide not only has an anxiolytic effect but also provides analgesic and sedative effects. This form of sedation involves the patient inhaling a mixture of nitrous oxide and oxygen through a nasal mask. Nitrous oxide sedation is widely used in dentistry because of its effectiveness in reducing anxiety and promoting relaxation during dental procedures.

"Nitrous oxide sedation is widely used in dentistry because of its effectiveness in reducing anxiety and promoting relaxation during dental procedures." (Kilicaslan, Cengiz, & Gurbuz, 2020)

Another type of hypnotic anesthesia used in dentistry is oral sedation, which involves the use of sedative drugs. Triazolam, for example, is a commonly used sedative that provides a pleasant sedative effect and helps to calm patients during dental procedures. It has anxiolytic properties and can induce an- terograde amnesia. There are several oral sedative and anxiolytic drugs available that have been developed to help reduce anxiety and promote relaxation in dental patients.

Intravenous sedation, also known as conscious sedation, is another hypnotic anesthesia commonly used in dentistry. This type of sedation involves the administration of sedative drugs through an intravenous route. Propofol, for example, is an ideal sedative anesthetic in dentistry due to its fast-acting nature and short half-life. Conscious sedation enhances the analgesic control provided by local anesthesia and helps patients achieve a state of mild hypnosis, relaxation, comfort and disengagement. Other medications, such as fentanyl, can also be used in intravenous sedation to provide analgesia and anesthesia. Intravenous conscious sedation, when combined with local anesthesia, allows for a comfortable and painless dental experience.

Preparation of the patient for hypnotic anesthesia

Preparation of the patient for hypnotic anesthesia in dentistry involves several important steps. The first step is the evaluation of the subject and review of his or her medical history. This is crucial to identify any underlying medical conditions or medications that may affect the administration of hypnotic anesthesia. Dental anxiety is a common phenomenon that significantly influences oral health status, making patient management during dental care challenging. Therefore, it is critical to assess anxiety levels and address any concerns that may exist prior to the procedure.

Communication and obtaining informed consent are vital aspects of preparing the patient for hypnotic anesthesia. The dentist should clearly explain the procedure, its benefits and any potential risks or side effects. This ensures that the patient is fully informed and can make an informed decision about his or her treatment. Informed consent is a legal and ethical requirement that protects both the patient and the dentist, ensuring that the subject understands the procedure and its implications.

In addition to communication and consent, providing pre-procedure instructions and fasting guidelines is crucial to prepare for hypnotic anesthesia. The patient should be given clear instructions on what to expect before, during and after the procedure. This includes fasting guidelines, as certain dental procedures may require the patient to refrain from eating or drinking for a specific period of time. Following these instructions helps ensure the safety and efficacy of hypnotic anesthesia during the dental procedure.

Administration of hypnotic anesthesia in dental practice

The administration of hypnotic anesthesia in dental practice requires careful monitoring of vital signs and ensuring patient safety throughout the procedure. It is crucial to continuously assess heart rate, blood pressure, and oxygen saturation levels to detect possible complications or adverse reactions [33]. This monitoring allows precise adjustment of hypnotic medication doses to maintain the desired level of sedation while ensuring patient comfort and safety. By closely monitoring vital signs, dental professionals can provide effective anesthesia and minimize the risks associated with sedation.

Dosing and titration of sedative medications play a key role in achieving the appropriate level of sedation for dental procedures. The choice of sedative medications and their dosages should be based on medical history, age and individual needs. Proper titration of sedative medications ensures that patients remain in a relaxed and comfortable state throughout the dental procedure.

Conscious sedation, which involves the administration of sedative medications to eliminate or reduce fear and anxiety in patients, is another effective technique used in dental procedures. These techniques allow for a more comfortable and stress-free dental experience for patients, particularly those with dental phobia or anxiety.

On the other hand, there is the option of using hypnotic suggestions within the trance state to generate the sensation of anesthesia without the use of drugs or by enhancing low doses of drugs to increase their duration or deepen their effect. An example to achieve the best benefit from hypnotic anesthesia is to provide the patient with suggestions to visualize that his jaw or the area to be worked on feels numb or numb, numb and numb, also using some analogy as a support (e.g. when holding an ice cube in his hand). In another way, hypnotic trance can be used to achieve a painless local dental anesthesia technique with total comfort for the patient and the clinician thanks to the dissociation that occurs while the subject is in trance and correctly using the refuge of the safe place.

Based on this, there are multiple benefits of the use of hypnotic trance in the application of both conventional hypnotic anesthesia and the previously mentioned using anesthetic suggestions in trance. The patient is able to be attended relaxed and safe, and the clinician works with greater confidence and certainty that the patient is comfortable and anesthetized.

Potential risks and complications of hypnotic anesthesia

A potential risk of hypnotic anesthesia in dentistry is the occurrence of allergic reactions and side effects. Allergic reactions to dental anesthesia may manifest as anaphylactic shock, urticaria, edema, pruritus, lacrimation or rhinitis. Although these reactions are rare, they can still occur and pose a risk to patients. In addition, there may be minor side effects associated with dental anesthesia, such as nausea or dizziness, which have an incidence rate of approximately 4.5%. It is important for dentists to be aware of these possible allergic reactions and side effects and take appropriate measures to minimize the risk to patients.

Another possible complication of hypnotic anesthesia is respiratory depression and airway compromise. Certain hypnotic drugs used in anesthesia can cause respiratory depression, which can lead to decreased oxygen levels and potentially compromise the airway. This highlights the importance of closely monitoring respiratory status during the administration of hypnotic anesthesia. Dentists should be prepared to intervene promptly in the event of any respiratory complications to ensure patient safety.

Drug interactions and contraindications are also important considerations when using hypnotic anesthesia in dentistry. Some patients may have existing medical conditions or be taking medications that may interact with the hypnotic drugs used in anesthesia. These interactions can potentially lead to adverse effects and complications. Dentists should carefully review the medical history and medication list to identify possible contraindications or drug interactions before administering hypnotic anesthesia. This thorough evaluation will help ensure the safe and effective use of hypnotic anesthesia in dental procedures.

Protocols and safety guidelines for hypnotic anesthesia

One of the key issues in ensuring the safety of hypnotic anesthesia in dentistry is the training and certification requirements for dental professionals. Anesthesiology is a specialized branch of medicine dedicated to pain relief and patient care during surgical procedures [39]. Dental professionals who wish to administer hypnotic anesthesia must undergo comprehensive training and obtain the necessary certifications to ensure that they have the necessary knowledge and skills to safely administer and monitor anesthesia. This training includes learning specific techniques for inducing and maintaining hypnosis, as well as understanding the potential risks and complications associated with hypnotic anesthesia. By meeting these training and certification requirements, dental professionals can ensure that they are well prepared to provide safe and effective hypnotic anesthesia to their patients.

Another crucial aspect of safety protocols for hypnotic anesthesia in dentistry is emergency preparedness and equipment maintenance. Dental professionals must be equipped to handle any emergencies that may arise during the administration of hypnotic anesthesia. This includes having emergency medications, such as reversal agents, readily available. In addition, regular maintenance and qualibration of anesthesia equipment is essential to ensure its proper functioning and accuracy. By being prepared for emergencies and maintaining their equipment, dental professionals can ensure the safety and well-being of their patients during the hypnotic anesthesia procedure.

Documentation and legal considerations are also important factors in ensuring the safety of hypnotic anesthesia in dentistry. Dental practitioners should keep detailed records of the hypnotic anesthesia procedure, including medications administered, vital signs monitored and any adverse events or complications that occur. This documentation not only serves as a reference for future treatments, but also ensures compliance with legal and regulatory requirements. By maintaining accurate and complete documentation, dental professionals can demonstrate their compliance with safety protocols and provide evidence of the quality of care provided during the hypnotic anesthesia procedure.

Case studies and success stories of hypnotic anesthesia in dentistry

Hypnotic anesthesia in dentistry has elicited positive comments and testimonials from patients, highlighting their satisfaction with this alternative approach to traditional anesthesia. Patients who have undergone dental procedures with hypnotic anesthesia reported feeling relaxed, calm and comfortable throughout the process. This high level of patient satisfaction demonstrates the effectiveness of hypnotic anesthesia in providing a positive dental experience. Through the use of hypnosis techniques, the patients reported feeling dentists can create a relaxing and calm environment, leading to better outcomes and overall patient satisfaction.

One of the significant advantages of hypnotic anesthesia is its successful management of dental phobia and anxiety. Dental phobia is a severe form of dental anxiety that can lead to irrational fear and avoidance of dental visits. Hypnotic anesthesia has been found to be particularly effective in reducing anxiety levels and helping patients overcome their dental fears. By inducing a state of deep relaxation, hypnosis allows them to feel more comfortable during dental procedures and ultimately improves their overall dental experience. This successful management of dental phobia and anxiety contributes to better oral health outcomes and encourages patients to seek regular dental care.

Hypnotic anesthesia has also been used successfully in the performance of complex dental procedures. Case studies have demonstrated the efficacy of hypnotic anesthesia in procedures such as dental extractions or maxillofacial surgeries of different types. By inducing a state of deep relaxation and reducing pain perception, hypnotic anesthesia allows dentists to perform complicated and lengthy procedures with ease. This alternative approach to anesthesia provides a viable option for patients who may have contraindications to traditional anesthesia methods. The use of hypnotic anesthesia in dentistry has expanded the treatment possibilities for patients with complex dental needs, ensuring their comfort and safety throughout the procedure.

Challenges and limitations of hypnotic anesthesia in dentistry

One of the challenges of using hypnotic anesthesia in dentistry is the variability of the individual patient and the response to sedation. Each patient may have a different level of susceptibility to hypnosis, making it difficult to predict the effectiveness of hypnotic anesthesia in achieving the desired level of sedation and analgesia. In addition, some patients may have underlying medical conditions or medications that may affect their response to sedation, further complicating the use of hypnotic anesthesia in dental procedures. Therefore, it is crucial that dental professionals carefully evaluate each patient's medical history and individual factors before deciding on the appropriateness of hypnotic anesthesia.

Another limitation of hypnotic anesthesia in dentistry is cost and insurance or health plan coverage considerations. While these may cover general anesthesia for certain dental procedures, hypnotic anesthesia may not always be included in the coverage. This may place a financial burden on patients who require hypnotic anesthesia for their dental treatment. In addition, the availability of trained professionals experienced in the administration of hypnotic anesthesia may be limited, especially in certain geographic areas. This lack of accessibility may further hinder the widespread use of hypnotic anesthesia in dentistry.

Finally, there have been concerns regarding the safety of dental procedures under any form of anesthesia, including hypnotic anesthesia. Although hypnotic anesthesia is generally considered safe when administered by trained practitioners, there is always a small risk of complications associated with sedation. These risks should be carefully weighed against the potential benefits of using hypnotic anesthesia in dental procedures. In addition, there may be certain dental procedures that are not suitable for hypnotic anesthesia because of their complexity or duration. Therefore, it is important for dental professionals to carefully assess the suitability of hypnotic anesthesia on a case-by-case basis, considering the specific needs and circumstances of each patient.

ANALGESIA HYPNOTIC

Introduction to hypnotic analgesia in dentistry

Hypnotic analgesia is a technique used in dentistry to control pain and discomfort during dental procedures. It involves inducing a state of deep relaxation and focused attention on the patient, allowing them to experience a reduced perception of pain. Pain management is of utmost importance in dentistry, as dental procedures can often be associated with significant discomfort and anxiety for patients. Hypnotic analgesia serves as an adjunct to chemical anesthesia and improves pain control during dental treatments. It has several applications within the dental field, ranging from relieving patient anxiety to providing analgesia. By using hypnotic techniques, dental professionals can help create a more comfortable and positive experience.

The role of hypnotic analgesia in dental procedures is to help patients achieve a state of relaxation and reduce their perception of pain. This can be achieved through various hypnotic phenomena, which include dissociation, sensory disturbances and anesthesia. The use of hypnosis in dentistry has been especially modeled to control neurophysiological and dental markers, ensuring optimal pain management. Studies have shown that hypnosis can be an effective alternative measure to control anxiety and pain in dental treatment. It may be particularly beneficial for patients who may fear dental procedures or who cannot tolerate traditional forms of anesthesia. By incorporating hypnotic analgesia techniques, dental professionals can provide a more comfortable and less stressful experience.

Hypnotic analgesia in dentistry offers an alternative approach to pain management, reducing dependence on traditional analgesic medications. This can be especially beneficial for patients who may have restrictions, contraindications or sensitivities to certain analgesics. The efficacy of hypnotic analgesia can be assessed using procedures such as the Cold Pressor Test (CPT), which allows the evaluation of different pain control treatments, including hypnotic analgesia. The increasing use of hypnosis in dentistry highlights its effectiveness in helping them undergo dental treatment with reduced pain and anxiety. By incorporating hypnotic analgesia techniques into dental practices, dental professionals can provide a more holistic, patient-centered approach to pain management.

How hypnotic analgesia works

Hypnotic analgesia in dentistry works by inducing a hypnotic state. This state of focused attention and increased suggestibility allows the patient to enter a deep state of relaxation, which helps to neutralize the nervousness and anxiety associated with procedures.

dental. However, it is important to note that the hypnotic state is only occasionally and selectively induced, and not everyone is a suitable candidate for this technique. Dentists who regularly use hypnosis in their clinical practices employ techniques such as distraction, reframing, and imagery suggestions to induce the hypnotic state and facilitate analgesia. The use of hypnosis has been found to be particularly useful in pediatric dentistry, where it can help to effectively manage dental anxiety and dental phobia.

During the hypnotic state, suggestions and imagery are used to enhance the analgesic effect. Dentists guide patients to imagine and visualize men- tally pleasant and relaxing images or scenarios, which helps to divert their attention from pain stimuli. By focusing on positive and calming suggestions, the patient's perception of pain is altered, leading to a reduction in pain intensity. This technique of using suggestions and imagery is an integral part of hypnotic analgesia in dentistry and contributes to the overall effectiveness of the treatment.

Activation of pain-modulating brain pathways is another mechanism through which hypnotic analgesia acts. Studies have shown that hypnosis can modulate pain perception by activating endogenous pain control systems in the brain. This involves activation of opioid receptors at both the spinal and supraspinal levels, resulting in analgesic effects. By harnessing the power of the brain's pain modulation pathways, hypnotic analgesia provides a nonpharmacologic approach to pain management in dentistry.

Benefits of hypnotic analgesia in the following situations
dentistry

One of the significant benefits of using hypnotic analgesia in dentistry is the reduction of anxiety and fear in patients. Dental anxiety is a common phenomenon that can significantly affect the dental care experience. Many dentists who incorporate hypnosis as a supportive technique report that they can alleviate the pain and fear experienced by their patients, particularly in anxiety-provoking situations. By inducing a state of deep relaxation and calmness through hypnosis, patients may feel calmer and more comfortable during dental procedures, leading to a more positive dental experience.

Another advantage of hypnotic analgesia in dentistry is the minimization of the need for traditional anesthesia. Traditional anesthetic techniques, such as the administration of local anesthetics like lidocaine, can sometimes be associated with discomfort or adverse effects. By incorporating hypnotic analgesia, dentists can reduce the dose and modulate the duration of anesthesia, minimizing the potential for toxicity and adverse reactions. This not only provides a safer approach to pain management, but also allows for a more personalized and individualized treatment plan for each patient.

Hypnotic analgesia in dentistry has also been found to contribute to faster recovery and reduce postoperative pain. By using hypnosis techniques, dentists can help control neu- rophysiological and dental markers, leading to better pain management and a more efficient recovery process. In addition, the administration of analgesics before, during and after surgery can further enhance the analgesic and pain-relieving effects of surgery.

reduce pain and inflammation. This comprehensive approach to pain management can result in faster recovery time and a more comfortable postoperative experience for patients.

Hypnotic techniques used in practice dental

One of the hypnotic techniques used in dental practices is guided imagery. Guided imagery involves using the power of the imagination to create a relaxing and pleasurable mental image that helps distract the patient from dental procedures and reduces anxiety. By focusing on the relaxing image, one can experience a sense of relaxation and comfort during their dental appointments. This technique has been found to be effective in reducing dental anxiety and pain. Dentists can guide patients through visualizations that transport them to calm and serene environments, allowing them to feel more comfortable during dental procedures.

Deep relaxation techniques are another form of hypnotic intervention used in dentistry. These techniques aim to induce a state of deep relaxation similar to sleep. By helping patients achieve a state of deep relaxation, dentists can relieve anxiety and create a more comfortable dental experience. This technique involves guiding them through relaxation exercises that focus on deep breathing, progressive muscle relaxation and mindfulness. Deep relaxation techniques can help patients feel calmer and more comfortable, reducing their perception of pain and discomfort during dental procedures.

Dentists often use affirmations and suggestions positive ways to help patients manage anxiety and pain, thus creating a more positive dental experience. Positive affirmations and suggestions can also help patients to divert their attention away from pain and discomfort, allowing them to better tolerate dental procedures. This technique is often used in combination with other hypnotic interventions to improve the overall effectiveness of pain management in dentistry.

Training and certification for dentists in hypnotic analgesia

Adequate training and certification in hypnotic analgesia are crucial for dentists to ensure the safe and effective use of these techniques in dental practice. As with any medical intervention, it is essential that dentists have the necessary knowledge and skills to administer hypnotic analgesia appropriately. The International Society of Hypnosis emphasizes the importance of disseminating the scientifically supported use of hypnosis in various fields, including dentistry. Dentists properly trained and certified in hypnotic analgesia can provide their patients with a safe and effective alternative to traditional methods of pain management.

The integration of hypnotic techniques into dental education is an important step in ensuring that future dentists are equipped with the skills necessary to use these techniques in their practice. By incorporating hypnotic analgesia training into dental curricula, dental schools can prepare their students to provide comprehensive care to their patients. This integration can help dentists address patient anxiety and phobia, promoting a sense of relaxation and comfort during dental procedures.

Dentists have access to several resources and organizations that offer training in hypnotic analgesia. These resources can provide the knowledge and skills necessary to incorporate hypnotic techniques into your practice. Organizations such as the American Society of Clinical Hypnosis and the International Society of Hypnosis offer training programs and workshops specifically designed for dentists. In addition, dental schools may offer continuing education courses or seminars on hypnotic analgesia. By taking advantage of these resources, dentists can expand their skill set and provide their patients with safe and effective alternative methods of pain management.

Case studies and success stories of hypnotic analgesia in dentistry

Hypnotic analgesia in dentistry has attracted attention for its potential to provide effective pain management during various dental procedures. Patient experiences with hypnotic analgesia have shown promising results in terms of pain reduction and overall satisfaction. Case studies have demonstrated the successful application of hypnotic anesthesia as the sole procedure for analgesia in dental extractions. In addition, hypnosis has been used to relax patients and relieve anxiety, leading to a more comfortable dental experience. Psychophysiological evidence supports the idea that hypnotic analgesia actively inhibits pain through various systems. Concrete patient experiences highlight the potential of hypnotic analgesia as a valuable tool in dental practice.

The use of hypnosis, along with other techniques such as distraction, topical anesthesia, and nitrous oxide, has been found to be effective in minimizing pain and discomfort.

during dental procedures. In addition, hypnosis has been explored as a possible alternative to conventional analgesics for acute dental and maxillofacial pain. These success stories highlight the versatility of hypnotic analgesia for pain control in different dental treatments.

In addition to immediate pain relief, hypnotic analgesia offers long-term benefits and high patient satisfaction. Those who undergo hypnosis during dental procedures report minimal or no pain perception, leading to improved communication between the dentist and patient. Improved communication contributes to optimal treatment outcomes and increased comfort for the individual as much as possible. In addition, hypnosis has been found to be particularly useful in pediatric dentistry, as it addresses problems such as dental anxiety and dental phobia. For patients who may not respond well to traditional medical and dental treatments, hypnosis offers a valuable alternative. In general, the long-term benefits and high satisfaction associated with hypnotic analgesia make it a promising approach in dentistry.

Possible limitations and considerations of hypnotic analgesia in dentistry

Patient selection and suitability for hypnotic techniques should be carefully considered in dentistry. While hypnosis can provide considerable relief to patients with anxiety disorders and facilitate the dentist's work, it is important to assess the individual's psychological and physical suitability for this technique. Not all patients may be receptive to hypnotic suggestions, and certain conditions, such as psychosis or severe cognitive impairment, may contraindicate the use of hypnosis.

Dentists should evaluate each patient individually to determine if they are suitable candidates for hypnotic analgesia and also choose the correct techniques to use in each case.

Ethical considerations and informed consent are crucial when implementing hypnotic analgesia in dentistry. Informed consent is an essential aspect of ethical dental practice, as it ensures that patients are fully aware of the risks, benefits, and alternatives to any treatment modality, including hypnosis. Dentists should provide clear and complete information about the use of hypnosis, its potential outcomes, and any possible limitations or side effects. Patients should have the opportunity to ask questions and make an informed decision about whether to proceed with hypnotic analgesia.

Collaboration with other dental professionals in pain management is important when using hypnotic analgesia in dentistry. While hypnosis can be a valuable tool for pain management, it should not be used as the sole method of pain control in dental procedures. Dentists should work in collaboration with other dental professionals, such as anesthesiologists or pain specialists, to develop a comprehensive pain management plan that incorporates hypnosis along with other techniques, such as local anesthesia or pharmacologic interventions. This multidisciplinary approach ensures that patients receive the most effective and appropriate pain relief during dental procedures.

Future prospects and research in hypnotic analgesia for dentistry.

Advances in hypnotic techniques and technologies have paved the way for the future prospects of hypnotic analgesia for dentistry. While informal hypnotic methods, such as the use of comforting utterances, have shown some efficacy in the management of pain and anxiety in dental patients, further research and development in this field may lead to more specific and efficient hypnotic interventions. The use of hypno- sis as an adjunct in psychotherapy has already demonstrated positive results, indicating its potential in dental settings as well. Researchers are exploring the integration of hypnosis with virtual reality technology to reduce anxiety and pain in children during dental procedures. These advances in hypnotic techniques and technologies promise to improve patient experience and outcomes in dental practices.

Further research on the effectiveness and safety of hypnotic analgesia in dentistry is crucial for its integration into conventional dental practices. While there are references to the use of hypnosis in dentistry, there is a need for more comprehensive studies to establish accurate conclusions and guidelines for its application. Studies have examined the efficacy of hypnosis as an adjuvant in cognitive-behavioral treatment and pain management, but more research is needed to validate these findings and determine optimal protocols for hypnotic analgesia in dental procedures. In addition, research focusing on neurophysiological and dental markers associated with hypnosis may provide valuable information on its mechanisms of action and further improve its efficacy. With continued research, the safety and efficacy of hypnotic analgesia can be improved.

better understanding, leading to greater acceptance and integration into conventional dental practices.

The integration of hypnotic analgesia into conventional dental practices may revolutionize the way pain and anxiety are managed in dental patients. Hypnosis has already found applications within the dental field, ranging from relaxation techniques to analgesia. By incorporating hypnosis as part of routine dental care, dentists can create a more comfortable and positive experience. This can lead to greater patient sa- tisfaction and improved treatment outcomes. In addition, the use of hypnosis can potentially reduce the need for traditional pain management techniques, such as local anesthesia, in some cases. However, proper training and education of dental professionals in the use of hypnotic techniques is essential to ensure their safe and effective application. With the integration of hypnotic analgesia, dental practices can offer a holistic, patient-centered approach to pain management, improving the overall quality of dental care.

CONTROL OF THE ANXIETY

Dental anxiety is a common problem that affects a large number of people worldwide. According to the World Health Organization (WHO), between 60% and 90% of the world's population experiences dental anxiety at some point in their lives (WHO, 2012). This anxiety can have a significant impact on oral health and quality of life. Therefore, it is important that dental health professionals are familiar with dental anxiety management techniques and use them effectively in the management of dental anxiety.

Hypnosis is a technique that has long been used to control dental anxiety. It involves inducing a trance-like state in the patient, in which specific suggestions can be provided to reduce anxiety and enhance relaxation. Through various hypnotic techniques, an enormous variety of problems related to dental anxiety can be treated, such as fear of dental procedures, preoperative and postoperative anxiety, and habituation to dental appliances, among others.

This book reviews the scientific literature on hypnosis techniques for managing dental anxiety. The effects of hypnosis in the management of dental anxiety are discussed and information on its efficacy and safety is provided. Some specific hypnosis techniques that have been used successfully in the management of dental anxiety are also presented.

Effects of Hypnosis in the Management of Dental Anxiety

Hypnosis can have several beneficial effects in the management of dental anxiety. First, it can reduce anxiety and fear associated with dental procedures. According to Lynn and Kirsch (2006), "hypnosis can reduce dental anxiety and improve the patient's experience during dental procedures". Hypnosis involves inducing a trance-like state in the patient, in which specific suggestions can be provided that are aggravating to the patient, leading to a tranquil state of mind that helps reduce anxiety and improve relaxation.

Second, hypnosis can reduce pain associated with dental procedures. According to Elkins et al. (2015), "hypnosis can be an effective technique for reducing dental pain and improving the patient experience during dental procedures" (p. 12). That is, it can be used to reduce the pain associated with anesthesia and with dental procedures themselves.

Third, hypnosis can improve patient cooperation during dental procedures. According to Spiegel (1993), "hypnosis can improve cooperation during dental procedures, which can improve the quality of the dentist's work and reduce the duration of procedures."

Effectiveness and Safety of Hypnosis in the Dental Anxiety Management

Hypnosis has been shown to be effective in the management of dental anxiety in several clinical studies. According to Lynn and Kirsch (2006), "hypnosis is an effective technique for reduce dental anxiety and improve the patient experience during dental procedures". Elkins et al. (2015) also found that hypnosis was effective in reducing dental pain and improving patient experience.

In addition, hypnosis has been shown to be safe in the management of dental anxiety. According to Lynn and Kirsch (2006), "hypnosis is a safe technique to control dental anxiety and presents no risk to the patient's health". Hypnosis is non-invasive and does not require the use of medication, which makes it a safe, effective and economical technique for the management of dental anxiety.

Specific Hypnosis Techniques for the Dental Anxiety Management

There are several specific hypnosis techniques that have been used successfully in the management of dental anxiety. Some of these techniques are presented below:

1. Guided Imagery: A technique in which the patient is guided through a series of relaxing mental images. This may include images of a relaxing place, such as a beach or a forest, or images of a state of physical and mental relaxation. Guided imagery can be used to reduce anxiety and improve relaxation before and during dental procedures.

2. Anchoring: This is a technique in which the patient associates a positive emotional state with a physical signal, such as a word or gesture. For example, the patient may associate a feeling of relaxation with a specific word, such as "calm". Anchoring can be used to help the patient to

to regain a state of relaxation during dental procedures.

3. Reframing: A technique in which the patient's perspective on a problem or situation is changed. For example, the patient may be fearful of dental procedures due to a previous bad experience. By reframing, the patient can be guided to see the situation differently, which can reduce the anxiety associated with dental procedures.

4. Positive Suggestions: These are statements made to the patient during hypnosis to enhance confidence and relaxation. For example, the hypnotist may suggest that the patient feel relaxed and calm during dental procedures. Positive suggestions can be used to reduce anxiety and improve the patient's experience during dental procedures.

FOBIA DENTAL

Dental phobia, also known as dentophobia, is an extreme and irrational fear of going to the dentist's office. People with dental phobia may experience symptoms such as difficulty sleeping the night before a dental examination and increased nervousness. This fear can last for more than six months and is considered a phobia. Fear of going to the dentist is often caused by anxiety, and the idea that dental procedures will be painful or uncomfortable. It is important to understand the definition and symptoms of dental phobia in order to address and overcome this fear.

Several common causes contribute to the development of dental phobia. One of the most frequent causes is the traumatic dental experiences, especially during childhood [4]. Negative experiences, such as a painful procedure or a dentist who lacks empathy, can leave a lasting impact and create fear and anxiety toward dental visits. In addition, fear of pain, embarrassment or loss of control can also contribute to dental phobia. It is essential to recognize these common causes in order to provide appropriate support and care for people with dental phobia.

Psychological factors also play an important role in dental phobia. Ge- neralized psychological vulnerability, which refers to an individual's general susceptibility to anxiety and fear, may contribute to the development of dental phobia. Other psychological factors that may contribute to phobia include a history of other fears and psychological disorders. Understanding these psychological factors can help dental professionals adapt their approach and provide a supportive environment for patients with dental phobia.

Systematic Desensitization

A technique commonly used in hypnosis to overcome phobias is systematic desensitization. Systematic desensitization is a technique used in hypnosis and cognitive-behavioral therapy to treat phobias and other anxiety disorders. This technique is based on the idea that a person can overcome his or her phobia through gradual and controlled exposure to the source of his or her fear. The systematic desensitization technique used in hypnosis involves exposing the individual gradually and safely to the source of his or her fear while in a state of hypnosis.

In the case of dental phobia, an individual with a fear of dental procedures may begin by imagining himself in a dental environment without fear. The hypnotist can guide the individual through a series of instructions to visualize the details of the dental environment, such as the waiting room, dental chair, lighting and sounds. The hypnotist may also use relaxation techniques to help the individual remain calm and relaxed during the visualization.

Once comfortable visualizing the dental environment, the hypnotist can proceed to visualize increasingly invasive dental procedures while the patient remains in a state of hypnosis. For example, the individual may visualize a simple dental procedure, such as a dental cleaning, and then proceed to more invasive procedures, such as a dental extraction or oral surgery.

As the subject progresses through the visualization of dental procedures, the hypnotist can use suggestive techniques to help the subject remain relaxed and calm. For example, the hypnotist may suggest that you feel calm and relaxed during dental procedures and that you trust the dental professional who is assisting you.

Over time, this systematic desensitization technique can help decrease the fear response to dental procedures. By gradually exposing the individual to the source of his or her fear while in a state of hypnosis, the individual can be helped to develop a greater tolerance to dental procedures and overcome his or her dental phobia.

Cognitive Restructuring

Cognitive restructuring is a technique used in hypnosis and cognitive-behavioral therapy to treat phobias and other anxiety disorders. This technique focuses on changing the way the patient perceives and thinks about their dental phobia, with the aim of reducing their anxiety and fear associated with it.

Cognitive restructuring is based on Beck's (1976) cognitive theory, which holds that negative thoughts and beliefs can contribute to a person's anxiety and depression. According to Beck, people may have negative and distorted thought patterns that contribute to their anxiety and depression. Cognitive restructuring aims to identify and challenge these negative thought patterns and replace them with more realistic and positive thoughts.

During hypnosis, the hypnotist can guide the individual through a series of instructions to identify and challenge his or her negative thought patterns about dental procedures. The hypnotist can help the individual see the situation from a more realistic and positive perspective. For example, the hypnotist can help the individual understand that most dental procedures are painless and that advances in dental technology have made procedures more comfortable and less invasive than in the past.

According to the study by Vann et al. (2014), "cognitive restructuring has been used successfully to treat dental phobia in patients experiencing severe dental anxiety". Cognitive restructuring can be used in conjunction with other hypnosis techniques, such as systemic desensitization and progressive relaxation, to improve the experience

The aim is to reduce the patient's dental anxiety during dental procedures and to obtain an integral benefit for the patient.

Once the individual has identified his or her negative thought patterns and has begun to question them, the hypnotist can use suggestive techniques to help strengthen his or her new thinking about dental procedures. For example, the hypnotist may suggest that they feel calm and relaxed during dental procedures and that they trust the dental professional who is treating them.

Hypnotic Regression

Hypnotic regression is an advanced hypnosis technique that can be particularly useful in overcoming deep-seated phobias, including dental phobia. During a hypnotic regression, the hypnotist guides the individual through their memories to identify and address the source of their phobia. This technique is based on the theory that phobias may be caused by past traumatic events that are stored in the person's subconscious.

In the case of dental phobia, hypnotic regression may involve identifying a past traumatic event related to dental care, such as a bad experience at the dentist or severe pain during a dental procedure. Once this event is identified, the hypnotist can work with the individual to change his or her perception of the event and lessen its emotional impact. For example, the hypnotist may help the individual visualize the event in a more tolerable and positive way, or may use suggestive techniques to help the individual release his or her fear and anxiety associated with the event. An example of this is to modify within the hypnotic visualization who the treating dentist is and replace him or her with a character that the patient finds pleasant or someone he or she trusts.

It is important to note that hypnotic regression is a complex and potentially emotional technique that should be performed by an experienced hypnosis practitioner. According to the study by Lynn et al. (2015), "hypnotic regression is an advanced technique that should be used with caution and only by well-trained and experienced hypnotists". The hypnotist should be experienced in identifying and addressing past traumatic events, and should be trained to help the individual process and release any unpleasant emotions that may arise during hypnotic regression, so psychologists or psychiatrists specialized in the technique are generally recommended. Based on this, it is important to consider that the odontologist should know how to initially handle possible traumatic events that may surface during the hypnotic experience and also duly refer and complement what has been done with a hypnotherapist psychologist to effectively treat the patient's afflictions.

It should be noted that, in our experience, this tool is the most effective and has permanent results over time.

Positive Suggestion

Positive suggestion is a hypnosis technique used to promote beneficial attitudes and behaviors. During hypnosis, the hypnotist may give positive suggestions to help alleviate fear and anxiety associated with dental care. Positive suggestion is based on the theory that the subconscious can be influenced by positive affirmations and suggestions, which can lead to positive changes in a person's behavior and attitude.

In the context of dental phobia, the hypnotist may use positive suggestion to help the individual to feel more relaxed and comfortable during dental procedures. For example, the hypnotist may suggest that you feel calm and relaxed in the dental chair, that you feel as if you are in a nice, safe place, or that you imagine a calm, relaxing place during the procedure. Positive suggestion can also be used to help you feel more comfortable with the dentist and to gain confidence in his or her professionalism and skill.

According to the study by Elkins et al. (2007), "positive suggestion can be a useful tool for relieving anxiety and pain associated with dental procedures". Positive suggestion can be used in combination with other hypnosis techniques, such as progressive relaxation and systematic desensitization, to improve the patient's experience and reduce dental anxiety.

REFLEX CONTROL EMETIC REFLEX CONTROL

The emetic reflex, also known as the gag reflex, is a natural protective mechanism of the body that helps prevent choking or ingestion of harmful substances. It is activated when a stimulus comes into contact with the back of the throat or the base of the tongue. The gag reflex is present in everyone to some extent, but some people may have an overactive gag reflex, which can pose challenges during dental procedures. This reflex can be triggered by several factors, including physical contact of dental instruments or materials with the sensitive areas of the mouth and throat, as well as psychological factors such as anxiety and fear. Understanding the emetic reflex and its triggers is crucial for dental professionals to effectively manage and address this problem during dental treatment.

Gag reflex management is of utmost importance in the field of dentistry to ensure patient comfort and safety during dental procedures. An exacerbated gag reflex can significantly hinder the progress of dental treatments and can even lead to avoidance of necessary dental care. Dental professionals can employ various techniques to help alleviate the gag reflex, such as the use of topical anesthetics to numb sensitive areas of the mouth, distraction techniques to divert the patient's attention, or relaxation techniques to reduce anxiety. It is essential that dentists have open communication with their patients to understand their individual triggers and develop personalized strategies to manage the emetic reflex effectively].

In some cases, the emetic reflex can be particularly difficult to manage, such as in patients receiving chemotherapy or in people with conditions such as cyclic vomiting syndrome. Chemotherapy-induced nausea and vomiting (CINV) is a common side effect of cancer treatment and can significantly affect patients' oral health and well-being. Dental professionals should collaborate with other health care providers to develop integrated treatment plans that take into account the unique needs and challenges of these patients. By understanding and addressing the emetic reflex, dental professionals can provide more comfortable and successful dental experiences for their patients, ultimately improving overall oral health outcomes.

Systematic Desensitization

Systematic desensitization may be useful for patients who anticipate the emetic reflex during certain dental procedures, such as taking impressions.

The patient is subjected to a gradual and controlled exposure to the situation that causes the emetic reflex. In the case of dental impression-taking, this could involve gradual exposure to the sensation of having a dental mold in the mouth. In a state of hypnosis, the patient can visualize the dental procedure in a safe and calm manner, which may help to decrease the intensity of the emetic reflex on future dental visits.

It is important to keep in mind that systematic desensitization should be performed by a professional experienced in cognitive-behavioral therapy and hypnosis, and should also be trained to help the patient to process and release any unpleasant emotions that may arise during the therapy.

Systematic desensitization is based on the associative learning theory, which suggests that emotional responses can be learned and unlearned through gradual exposure to stimuli that provoke the emotional response. With systematic desensitization, the goal is to help the patient learn to manage and control his or her emotional response to the situation that causes his or her anxious response or emetic reflex trigger.

Physiological Response Control

Physiological response control is a technique used to help people control their physical responses, such as the emetic reflex. Hypnosis can be a powerful tool for physiological response control, as it can help to change the patient's mindset and thus influence their physical responses.

The connection between the mind and the body is intrinsic, and studies have shown that stress and anxiety can trigger physical responses in the body, such as the emetic reflex. Hypnosis can help reduce stress and anxiety by inducing a state of relaxation and calmness in the patient. This can be achieved through visualization and suggestion. The hypnotist can guide the patient through a series of instructions to help him or her reach a state of deep relaxation. Once the patient is in a state of deep relaxation, the dentist can guide the patient through a visualization of the procedure that causes the emetic reflex, which can help the patient learn to control his or her physical response to the particular situation.

It is important to keep in mind that hypnosis is not an appropriate technique for everyone. Some people may have certain medical or psychological conditions that could make hypnosis inappropriate or dangerous. Therefore, it is important that anyone considering hypnosis as a treatment for physiological response control consult with a mental health professional experienced in this technique.

Positive Suggestion

The study by Lang et al. (2000) found that positive suggestion can be effective in reducing anxiety and improving quality of life in patients with chronic illness. In this study, patients who received positive suggestion reported significantly lower levels of anxiety and an increase in their quality of life.

Regarding positive suggestion for dental procedures, the study by Kwek et al. (2015) found that positive su- ggestion can significantly reduce dental anxiety in patients experiencing severe dental fear and anxiety. In this study, patients who received

The patients with positive suggestion prior to a dental procedure reported significantly lower levels of dental anxiety than patients who did not receive the technique.

As an example of an intervention, during the state of hypnosis, the hypnosis-trained dentist may suggest to the patient that he or she has total control over his or her body, including his or her emetic reflex. For example, he may say something like, "You are a very strong and capable person, and you can control your body through your mind. You can control your emetic reflex and keep it under control at all times. If you feel the reflex starting to appear, you can take a deep breath and relax to control it.

It may also suggest that dental procedures will be a calm, nausea-free experience. For example, the hypnotist may say something like, "When you go to the dentist, you will feel relaxed and calm. You will not feel nauseous or uncomfortable during the procedure. Your mind and body are at peace and in harmony, and you can trust that everything will be fine.

Visualization

Visualization is an effective technique used in hypnosis to help patients control their physical and emotional responses. Visualization can be particularly useful in controlling the emetic reflex.

During the hypnotic state, the hypnotist can guide the patient through a series of instructions to help the patient reach a state of deep relaxation. Once the patient is in a state of deep relaxation, the dentist can guide the patient through a visualization of the procedure that causes the emetic reflex.

The patient may visualize his emetic reflex as an object or an image that can be manipulated. For example, he may visualize his reflex as a dial that can be turned downward, which reduces the intensity of the reflex, a button or switch that can be turned on or off that can be extrapolated to the reflex. Or you can visualize your reflex as a dark cloud that dissipates with each deep, relaxing breath.

Visualization helps the patient learn to control his or her physical response to the emetic reflex by allowing the patient to visualize the emetic reflex as something that can be controlled and manipulated. By visualizing his or her emetic reflex in this way, the patient can learn to control his or her physical response to the emetic reflex effectively.

BRUXISM

Bruxism, which is characterized by grinding, clenching or gnashing of the teeth, can have several causes. Psychological and emotional factors are among them. Stress and anxiety are considered important contributors to bruxism, especially during wakefulness. Inadequately managed stress can manifest itself through bruxism. In addition, bruxism has been linked to negative emotions such as anger, anxiety, frustration and stress. During sleep, emotional stress can be processed and manifested through bruxism. Therefore, it is important to properly address and manage stress and anxiety to prevent or reduce bruxism.

In addition to psychological and emotional factors, there are physical and dental factors that may contribute to the development of bruxism. Improper alignment of the teeth, sleep disorders and muscle sensitivity are some of the physical causes that can trigger bruxism. Ear pain, headache and neck pain may also be related to bruxism. Therefore, it is important to address any underlying physical or dental problems to effectively treat bruxism.

In addition to psychological, emotional and physical factors, it has also been observed that bruxism may have genetic and hereditary causes. Some studies suggest that certain neurotransmitters and their pathways, such as dopamine and gamma-aminobutyric acid (GABA), may be involved in the development of bruxism. In addition, genetic and hereditary factors may increase the predisposition to develop bruxism. However, it is important to keep in mind that bruxism is a multifactorial condition and that the interaction of several factors may contribute to its occurrence. In conclusion, bruxism can have a variety of causes, including psychological and emotional factors, physical and dental factors, as well as genetic and hereditary factors. To effectively treat bruxism, it is important to address and treat the underlying factors that contribute to its development.

Hypnosis has been shown to be effective in reducing the symptoms of bruxism and preventing tooth wear. Studies have found that hypnosis can help reduce involuntary tension of the jaw muscles by reducing nerve tension. Traditional treatments for bruxism, such as occlusal planes or splints, have been successful in preventing tooth wear. However, hypnosis offers a noninvasive alternative that targets the root cause of bruxism. In addition, biofeedback and relaxation techniques, including self-hypnosis, have also shown promise in the management of bruxism. By incorporating hypnosis into a comprehensive treatment plan, individuals with bruxism can experience symptom relief and protect their oral health.

Untreated bruxism can have serious consequences on oral health. One of the most significant consequences is tooth wear, which can be more aggressive when bruxism is associated with sleep. Continuous grinding and clenching of the teeth can lead to enamel erosion, tooth sensitivity and even tooth fractures. In addition, bruxism can also cause secondary symptoms such as insomnia, headaches, earaches and neck pain. It is important to address bruxism to prevent further damage to the teeth and alleviate the associated symptoms. While there is no foolproof treatment for bruxism, measures such as hypnosis can be taken to control the condition and minimize its impact on oral health.

Understanding the Role of Hypnosis in the Management of Bruxism

Hypnosis, also known as hypnotherapy, is a therapeutic technique that consists of inducing a heightened state of consciousness, or trance, to facilitate positive changes in behavior and mentality. Contrary to popular belief, the main objective of hypnotherapy is not to manipulate the patient, but to provide him with the tools he needs to regain control over his thoughts and actions. This technique has been used in various fields, including health care, to address a wide range of health problems. In the context of bruxism, hypnosis can play an important role in helping people control and manage teeth grinding and clenching.

Research and studies have shown that hypnosis can be an effective tool for controlling bruxism. One study explored the use of hypnosis to reduce teeth grinding and improve sleep quality in people with bruxism. The results indicated that hypnosis can be beneficial in controlling the symptoms of bruxism. In addition, hypnosis has been recognized as a complementary therapy in psychotherapy, and its efficacy in managing stress-related behaviors, such as teeth grinding, has been acknowledged. In addition, individuals can access recorded hypnosis sessions online to specifically address and treat bruxism.

While hypnosis has shown promise in the management of bruxism, it is important to keep in mind that its efficacy may vary from person to person. Some studies have reported positive results in the use of hypnosis to improve sleep bruxism, while others have found it to be less effective. In addition, hypnosis should be considered as part of a comprehensive treatment plan that may include other techniques such as psychoanalysis, progressive relaxation and self-management. It is essential to consult with a qualified health professional or therapist who specializes in hypnosis to determine the most appropriate approach to controlling bruxism.

Deep Relaxation

Deep relaxation is an effective technique used in hypnosis to reduce tension and stress in the body and mind. In the context of bruxism treatment, hypnosis can be used to induce a state of deep relaxation before bedtime, which can help reduce the likelihood of clenching and grinding during sleep.

During hypnosis, the dentist can guide the patient through a series of instructions to help the patient reach a state of deep relaxation. Once the patient is in a state of deep relaxation, the hypnotist can guide the patient through a visualization or suggestion to release tension in the jaw and facial muscles.

The dentist may suggest to the patient to imagine that tension is gradually being released from the jaw and facial muscles, and that they are feeling a sense of relaxation and calm. The specialist may also suggest to the patient to imagine that they are sleeping deeply and peacefully, without clenching or grinding their teeth.

By reducing tension in the jaw and facial muscles and promoting a state of deep relaxation, hypnosis can be effective in reducing the propensity to clench and grind the teeth during sleep.

Post-Hypnotic Suggestions

Post-hypnotic suggestions are a powerful tool in the management of unwanted behaviors such as bruxism. They are often used in combination with other hypnosis techniques to help individuals change their behavioral patterns in daily life.

Post-hypnotic suggestions are instructions given to an individual while in a state of hypnosis that have continuing effects after the hypnosis session has ended. They are based on the idea that the brain can learn new responses to specific stimuli, even in a state of sleep or subconsciousness. These ins- tructions can help individuals change their behavior at a subconscious level.

For example, in the context of bruxism, a post-hypnotic suggestion might be, "Whenever you feel your teeth begin to clench, your jaw muscles will automatically relax." This suggestion would be given while the individual is in a state of hypnosis. Subsequently, when the individual begins to clench the teeth during sleep, the jaw automatically relaxes in response to this tension.

Post-hypnotic suggestions can be highly customized to suit the patient's individual needs. For example, if a patient specifically associates bruxism with stressful situations, the post-hypnotic suggestion can be linked to the feeling of stress. In this case, the suggestion might be: "Every time you feel stress, you will notice the tension in your jaw and allow it to relax."

The power of post-hypnotic suggestions lies in their ability to bring about changes in behavior.

subconscious. By using post-hypnotic suggestions, individuals can work to reduce or eliminate bruxis- mo, even at times when they are not fully conscious, such as during sleep.

Also, it should be noted that the success of post-hypnotic su- gencies may vary from one individual to another. While some may experience a significant reduction in bruxism after one or two sessions, others may require several sessions before changes are observed. As with any treatment, it is essential to take an individualized approach and be willing to make adjustments as needed.

Visualization

Visualization is a highly effective technique in hypnosis and other types of therapy. This is because the mind can powerfully influence the body. In the context of bruxism, visualization can be a very useful tool.

During a hypnosis session, the dentist may guide the patient into a state of deep relaxation and then help the patient visualize an image or scene that represents jaw relaxation. For example, the practitioner might suggest that the patient imagine the jaw as a bundle of loose, relaxed cords. Or perhaps the patient could visualize a calm sea, with each wave reaching the shore representing further relaxation in the jaw.

Visualization can be even more effective when combined with post-hypnotic suggestions. For example, the dentist might suggest that when the patient goes to sleep, they will remember the image of the relaxed jaw or the calm sea, and that this image will help them keep the jaw relaxed while they sleep.

Hypnotic Regression

Hypnotic regression is a therapy technique that uses hypnosis to guide an individual through past experiences. This technique can be useful in treating problems such as bruxism that may have deep roots in past experiences or traumas.

Hypnotic regression is based on the idea that our past experiences, particularly traumatic or stressful ones, can significantly impact our current behavior. Sometimes these past events may be repressed or forgotten at the conscious level, but they can still influence our behavior at the subconscious level.

By using hypnosis to access these forgotten or repressed memories, a hypnotherapist can help an individual confront and process these experiences. This process can allow them to better understand how their past experiences are influencing their current behavior and give them the tools to change these behavioral patterns.

In the case of bruxism, an individual may have developed the habit of grinding his or her teeth in response to a stressful or traumatic situation. By using hypnotic regression to explore and understand these past experiences, the subject can begin to disassociate the stress or trauma from the need to grind his or her teeth. This can result in a significant reduction in bruxism.

In addition, hypnotic regression can provide a safe space for patients to confront and process past experiences that may be difficult to address in a conscious state. Hypnosis can help them enter into a state of deep relaxation and concentration, which can facilitate the process of reliving and processing these difficult experiences.

It is important to note that hypnotic regression should be performed by a trained hypnotherapist. This technique may involve confronting past experiences that may be emotionally difficult or traumatic. An experienced hypnotherapist can provide the support necessary to navigate these experiences safely and effectively.

In addition, the success of hypnotic regression may vary from person to person. Some individuals may find significant relief from bruxism after one or two sessions, while others may need several sessions to fully address the problem. In general, however, hypnotic regression can be a valuable tool in the treatment of bruxism, particularly when used in combination with other hypnosis techniques.

In the end, the most important thing is to work closely with a skilled mental health professional or hypnotherapist who can provide personalized therapy based on each individual's unique needs and circumstances. In this way, hypnosis techniques, including hypnotic regression, can be an effective way to treat bruxism and improve an individual's quality of life.

Self-hypnosis

Self-hypnosis is a powerful technique that can help people access their subconscious and make positive changes in their behavior and life in general. In the context of bruxism, self-hypnosis can be a particularly useful tool for relieving the tension of bruxism.

and stress, two factors that often contribute to teeth grinding and clenching.

By learning self-hypnosis techniques under the guidance of a qualified hypnotherapist, individuals can take active control of their own healing process. Instead of relying on medication or physical control measures, they can use the power of their mind to relieve the tension in their jaws and prevent bruxism.

The process of self-hypnosis usually involves entering a state of deep relaxation, often through controlled breathing exercises. Once this state of relaxation has been achieved, patients may begin to visualize images or scenes that help them relax and release tension in their jaws. This can be accompanied by the repetition of mantras or positive affirmations, such as "Every night, while I sleep, my jaw muscles relax and my teeth remain separated".

The key to success in self-hypnosis lies in repetition and consistency. As with any other skill, practice makes perfect. By regularly practicing self-hypnosis, individuals can strengthen the neural connections associated with relaxation and tension release, which over time can lead to a decrease in the incidence of bruxism.

Self-hypnosis can also be a valuable adjunct to other forms of treatment for bruxism. For example, it can be useful in combination with cognitive-behavioral therapy, which focuses on helping individuals identify and change negative thought patterns and behaviors. Together, these techniques can offer a complete solution to relieving bruxism.

In addition, self-hypnosis has the advantage of being a technique that they can practice on their own, in the comfort of their own home. This means that they can apply the techniques whenever they need to, for example, before going to bed to help prevent nighttime bruxism.

However, it is important to note that although autohypnosis can be a very effective technique, it is not a miracle cure and will not work for everyone. Some people may find more benefit from other treatment approaches. In addition, self-hypnosis should be learned with the help of a qualified professional to ensure that it is being performed safely and effectively.

Despite these considerations, for many people, self-hypnosis can be a valuable tool in the array of techniques available to treat bruxism. By offering a way to relieve tension and stress, it can help people achieve more peaceful nights of sleep and live healthier, happier lives.

Anchoring Technique

The anchoring technique is a method based on the principles of classical conditioning, where a particular response is associated with a specific stimulus. This technique, used in hypnosis therapy, can be especially useful in managing bruxism by linking a stimulus with a relaxation response.

To understand anchoring, it is useful to recall the famous experiment of Pavlov and his dogs. Pavlov noticed that, after a while, his dogs began to salivate at the sound of the bell that usually announced food. They had associated the sound of the bell with food, so their reaction was automatic and predictable. In the same way, the

Hypnotic anchoring can teach people to associate a specific stimulus with a relaxation response.

In bruxism therapy, an anchor can be any sensory stimulus: a sound, an image, a gesture or even a specific word. For example, the hypnotherapist could teach the patient to touch the thumb with the index finger each time he or she feels tension in the jaw or the onset of teeth clenching. This gesture would serve as an anchor.

During the hypnosis session, the hypnotherapist will guide the patient into a state of deep relaxation. Then, the hypnotherapist will associate the feeling of relaxation with the anchoring gesture. This can be done, for example, by saying something like: "Every time you touch your thumb with your index finger, you feel a deep and pleasant feeling of relaxation in your jaw". This instruction is repeated several times during hypnosis to reinforce the association between the anchor and the relaxation response.

With time and practice, the anchoring gesture will automatically trigger a relaxation response in the jaw whenever you feel the need to clench or grind your teeth. It is important to mention that, to be effective, anchoring must be practiced regularly, even after hypnosis sessions.

One of the advantages of the anchorage technique is that it provides the individual with a practical and easy-to-use tool that can help control bruxism in daily life. However, anchorage is not a magic cure, but a technique that can be very effective if practiced regularly and combined with other forms of therapy.

Ericksonian Hypnosis

Ericksonian hypnosis differs significantly from traditional direct hypnosis techniques in that instead of using direct commands, it is characterized by the use of metaphors, stories, symbols, and indirect suggestions to help people make changes at the subconscious level. Erickson believed that each individual has the inner resources necessary to solve his or her own problems and that the therapist's task is to help the client recognize and tap these resources.

In the context of bruxism, a hypnotherapist using Ericksonian techniques might use a variety of strategies to help the client reduce or eliminate clenching or grinding. For example, the therapist might tell a story about a character who learns to release tension in his or her body in healthy and effective ways, indirectly suggesting to the client new ways to manage the tension that may be contributing to bruxism. The practitioner might also use metaphors related to relaxation and tension release.

Another characteristic of Ericksonian hypnosis is its focus on the "here and now. Erickson believed that being present and focusing on current experiences can be especially helpful in overcoming problematic behavior patterns. In the case of bruxism, the specialist may guide the client to focus on the current sensations in his or her jaw and mouth, helping him or her to recognize any tension and explore ways to release that tension.

Ericksonian hypnosis is also characterized by its respect for the client and its ability to make changes. Erickson believed that each individual is unique and that there is no single "recipe" that works for everyone. Therefore, a

Ericksonian hypnotherapist will customize his or her approach to
to suit the customer's specific needs and objectives.

DECREASE OF BLEEDING

Hypnosis, as a technique used in dentistry, has gained recognition for its ability to reduce pain and improve the patient experience. Hypnosis is a state of focused attention and increased suggestibility, where people are more open to positive suggestions and can override their conscious mind. In the field of dentistry, hypnosis is used to help patients overcome anxiety, fear and phobia associated with dental procedures. By inducing a state of relaxation and calm, hypnosis can effectively neutralize nervousness and create a more comfortable environment for both the patient and the dentist. The use of hypnosis in dentistry has a long history and has evolved over time to become a valuable tool for improving patient outcomes.

The benefits of the use of hypnosis in dentistry are manifold. One significant advantage is the reduction of bleeding during dental procedures. While chemical anesthesia may cause some bleeding, hypnoanesthesia has been found to be associated with minimal bleeding. This may be attributed to the relaxation and control of physiologic responses achieved through hypnosis. By reducing stress and anxiety, hypnosis helps regulate blood flow and decreases the likelihood of excessive bleeding. In addition, hypnosis can facilitate pain control, allowing for a more comfortable and painless dental experience. The use of hypnosis in dentistry has been recognized as an alternative measure to control anxiety and pain in adult patients.

The use of hypnosis in oral treatment offers many advantages for both the patient and the dental professional. For the patient, hypnosis reduces the apprehension, fear and pain associated with dental procedures. It improves communication between the patient and the dentist, creating a more relaxed and cooperative environment. Hypnosis also helps patients undergo dental treatment in a more relaxed, fearless and pain-free manner. For the dental professional, hypnosis can enhance his or her ability to perform dental procedures effectively and efficiently. It can also contribute to a positive patient experience, leading to greater patient satisfaction and loyalty. Overall, the use of hypnosis techniques in dentistry has proven to be a valuable tool for decreasing bleeding, reducing anxiety, and improving the overall dental experience for both patients and dental professionals.

Visualization and Direct Suggestion

Visualization and direct suggestion are effective hypnosis techniques that can be used for a variety of purposes, including decreasing bleeding.

Visualization involves the patient imagining a scenario or situation in which the body is performing a desired function. In the case of decreased bleeding, a dentist may guide the patient to visualize that the blood vessels in the area of the procedure are constricting. The patient may be asked to imagine the process of blood vessel contraction, detailing each step of the process. As the patient visualizes this scenario, he or she can begin to influence the body's response at the physiological level.

Direct suggestion is another effective method in hypnosis. In this case, the practitioner provides instructions explicitly to the patient's subconscious mind. For example, the patient may be told, "Your body has the ability to control and minimize bleeding. Imagine that you are sending messages to the blood vessels in the affected area to constrict and reduce the flow of blood". In addition, suggestions can be made on the basis of analogies, for example, asking the patient to imagine that his or her blood vessels are water channels that have gates that can open or close and that he or she can regulate their flow.

It should be noted that although these techniques may be effective for some patients, not everyone responds in the same way to hypnosis. The success of these techniques depends largely on the individual's receptiveness to hypnosis and the hypnotherapist's ability to customize the approach to the patient's specific needs.

Relaxation and Stress Management

It is well known that stress and anxiety can have a significant impact on the body's physiology. Among the body's various responses to stress is vaso- constriction, the narrowing of blood vessels, which can contribute to increased bleeding. Therefore, learning to manage and reduce stress can be an effective strategy to decrease bleeding.

Hypnosis can be an effective means of helping patients manage stress and anxiety. During a hypnosis session, the dentist can guide the patient through deep breathing techniques and tranquil visualizations to promote a state of calm and relaxation.

Deep breathing techniques involve inhaling slowly and deeply through the nose, holding the breath for a few seconds and then exhaling slowly through the mouth. This process can help to slow down the heart rate and relax the body, thereby reducing the body's stress response.

Calm visualizations, on the other hand, involve the patient imagining themselves in a calm and peaceful place. This can help reduce anxiety and stress by promoting feelings of peace and tranquility.

In addition, the dentist may use suggestions for calm and relaxation. These suggestions may be things like "You feel completely calm and relaxed" or "Every breath you take makes you feel calmer and more relaxed." These suggestions, delivered while the patient is in a hypnotic state, can help promote greater relaxation and reduce stress and anxiety.

Therefore, through relaxation and stress control, hypnosis can be a useful tool to help control and reduce bleeding during and after dental procedures. However, it is important to note that hypnosis techniques should be administered by a trained professional to ensure their effectiveness and safety.

Hypnotic Anesthesia

Hypnotic anesthesia, or hypnotic analgesia, refers to the ability of hypnosis to reduce or eliminate the perception of pain. Through hypnotic suggestions, an individual can be guided to feel less pain or even no pain perception at all.

The ability of hypnosis to mitigate pain perception has been demonstrated in several investigations. For example, the study by Lang et al., published in the journal "Pain" in 2000, showed that patients undergoing interventional radiology procedures who received hypnosis reported significantly less pain and anxiety than those who did not receive hypnosis.

In addition, a meta-analysis by Patterson and Jensen, published in the Journal of Pain in 2003, examined the effects of hypnosis on pain relief in 18 separate studies. The analysis concluded that hypnosis can be an effective intervention for reducing pain in a variety of conditions.

In the context of dentistry, hypnotic anesthesia can be used to help patients manage pain during dental procedures. Through the use of hypnotic techniques, patients can learn to reduce their perception of pain, which can minimize the body's stress response, thereby reducing the risk of excessive bleeding.

It is important to note that although hypnotic anesthesia can be effective, it is not suitable for all patients or all procedures. It should be administered by a trained professional and used with caution, especially in more invasive or complex procedures.

Post-Hypnotic Suggestions

Post-hypnotic suggestions are an important technique in hypnosis and may be especially useful in the control of bleeding after dental surgery. These suggestions are provided during hypnosis and are intended to have an effect after the person has emerged from the hypnotic state.

The nature of these suggestions can vary widely, depending on the specific needs and goals of the patient. In the context of post-dental health monitoring, a post-hypnotic suggestion might involve instructing the patient to, after the intervention, the affected area will heal quickly and bleeding will be minimal. This suggestion is reinforced during the hypnotic state, establishing a link in the mind between the intervention and the response of rapid healing and minimal blood loss.

The goal of this post-hypnotic suggestion is to involve the subconscious mind in the healing process. Through hypnosis, the patient can be led to believe in his or her ability to control and minimize bleeding, and this belief can influence his or her actual physical response to the intervention.

It is important to keep in mind that post-hypnotic suggestions must be personalized for each individual, and it is essential that they be formulated in a way that is positive, beneficial and safe.

In addition, although hypnosis can be an effective tool for pain management and control of bleeding, it should not be used as a substitute for appropriate medical care. Patients should always follow the recommendations of their health care professionals regarding postoperative care and the management of any complications.

Ericksonian Hypnosis

Ericksonian hypnosis, also known as indirect hypnosis, was developed by Milton Erickson and is distinguished by its individual-centered approach and its use of metaphors, stories, and indirect innuendo to facilitate change.

In the context of bleeding control, a dentist using Ericksonian techniques might begin by establishing a state of deep relaxation and openness to the suggestions. Next, instead of giving di- rect suggestions, the therapist could tell a story or use a metaphor that relates to the diminishing flow of water, such as a stream that gradually transforms into a smooth, calm stream.

This metaphor serves as a form of direct communication with the subconscious mind, suggesting the idea that the bleeding can decrease and become a smoother, more controlled flow. The idea is that the patient's subconscious mind interprets this metaphor and applies it to the actual situation, leading to an actual decrease in bleeding.

An important element of Ericksonian hypnosis is that it respects the individuality of the patient and his or her own ability to solve problems. Therefore, the practitioner does not "instruct" the patient on what to do, but rather provides the tools and suggestions that allow the patient to find his or her own solution to the situation. This can be particularly effective in the management of physiological responses such as bleeding, as each person may have different ways of visualizing and understanding this process.

DISCOMFORT DURING CLEANING

Dental prophylaxis (scaling), also known as dental cleaning, is an integral component of oral health preservation. However, despite its undisputed importance, this procedure may cause discomfort in some patients. This feeling of discomfort may be particularly acute in individuals who experience dental sensitivity or in those who are prone to develop an aversion to dental tools. In these contexts, oral health professionals are challenged to provide effective dental care while minimizing patient discomfort to ensure a more tolerable experience and thereby increase adherence to future preventive and therapeutic procedures.

In this line, hypnosis has proved to be an effective method to alleviate these discomforts, transforming the dental encounter into a more pleasant experience. This technique, a non-invasive psychological intervention, works by modulating the patient's perception and emotional responses to the dental experience, which can lead to a decrease in the anticipation of pain and anxiety related to the treatment.

It is relevant to note that the implementation of certain technologies, such as ultrasound tools for dental cleaning, can potentially exacerbate anxiety or anticipation of discomfort in some patients. This possibility is especially pertinent in the case of individuals with acute hearing sensitivity. The characteristic sound emitted by ultrasound devices may cause stress or discomfort, which may ultimately negatively impact the patient's overall experience during the dental procedure.

In such situations, hypnosis emerges as an exceptionally useful tool capable of reducing the perception of discomfort during the procedure. By implementing hypnosis techniques, oral health professionals can help patients enter a state of deep relaxation, which can significantly change the perception of the sounds of the ultrasound tools and the overall level of discomfort associated with the dental procedure. Thus, hypnosis can be a valuable ally in modern dental practice, especially when it comes to optimizing the patient experience and improving the overall quality of dental care.

Hypnotic Induction and Relaxation

Progressive Relaxation: Before beginning the dental cleaning procedure, the dentist may guide the patient through a series of relaxation exercises. This could involve systematically tensing and relaxing different muscle groups in the body, starting from the feet and moving up to the head. This can help relieve physical tension and contribute to an overall sense of calm and relaxation.

Visualization: The dentist may ask the patient to imagine a place or situation that he or she finds particularly relaxing. It could be a quiet beach, a serene garden, or any other place that evokes a sense of peace. By keeping this image in mind during the dental procedure, the patient may feel that the experience is less stressful and more manageable.

Suggestion: In hypnosis, suggestion is a powerful tool. The dental health professional might suggest to the patient to feel a numbing sensation in the mouth, for example, or to perceive the sensations of the tooth cleaning in a different way, such as a numbing sensation in the mouth, or to perceive the sensations of the tooth cleaning in a different way, such as a numbing sensation in the mouth, for example.

tingling sensation instead of acute discomfort. This may change the patient's perception of the experience, making it less uncomfortable.

Noise management: For patients who are anxious about ultrasound tool noises, the dentist could use several techniques. For example, they could suggest that the sound of the tools is similar to the sound of ocean waves, a gentle rain or a friendly bee flying from flower to flower, or give a direct suggestion that the patient hears only the sound of the practitioner's voice and the other sounds fade or increasingly relax the patient. Alternatively, they could teach the patient deep breathing or mental focusing techniques to help divert his or her attention away from the noise.

Hypnotic Anesthesia

In the context of a dental cleaning, the dental professional could guide the patient through a process of relaxation and suggestion. First, relaxation techniques could be used to help the patient achieve a state of hypnosis. This could involve concentration on breathing, progressive muscle relaxation, or visualization of a calm and relaxed place.

Once the patient has reached a state of hypnosis, the dentist can begin to introduce suggestions that will help relieve pain and discomfort. For example, he might suggest to the patient that his mouth is beginning to feel numb and comfortable, similar to the sensation experienced with local anesthesia. You could reinforce this suggestion by describing the numb sensation in detail, or even suggesting that the patient cannot feel the dental tools in his or her mouth.

Visualization and Direct Suggestion

Visualization and direct suggestion are two hypnotic techniques that can be used to change the patient's perception of the dental cleaning experience.

In the case of visualization, the dentist might guide the patient through a process in which he or she imagines the tooth cleaning in a positive way. For example, the patient might be asked to visualize their teeth being gently cleaned, with each movement of the dental tool removing bacteria and leaving their teeth healthier and brighter. This visualization can help change the patient's perception of teeth cleaning from a potentially uncomfortable experience to a beneficial soothing experience.

In terms of direct suggestion, the dentist could provide positive and direct affirmations to the patient. These statements could be something like, "You will feel a soft, soothing sensation as we clean your teeth" or "Each movement of the dental tool brings you closer to having healthier, brighter teeth." These direct statements can help reinforce the positive perception of teeth cleaning in the patient's mind.

Post-Hypnotic Suggestions

Post-hypnotic suggestions are a fundamental part of many hypnosis procedures. These suggestions are given while the patient is in a hypnotic state and are designed to continue to have an effect after the patient has emerged from hypnosis.

In the context of a dental cleaning, the dentist may use post-hypnotic suggestions to help improve patient comfort and satisfaction after the cleaning.

procedure. For example, he or she might suggest that, once the dental cleaning is complete, the patient's teeth will feel extremely clean, fresh and comfortable. The practitioner might also suggest that any feelings of discomfort or sensitivity that the patient may have experienced during the cleaning will quickly diminish once the cleaning is complete.

In addition, post-hypnotic suggestions can be used to help the patient maintain good oral hygiene habits in the future. For example, the dentist might suggest that the patient will feel a strong desire to brush and floss regularly, or that he or she will find it easy to remember to make regular appointments for dental cleanings.

Distraction Techniques

Distraction techniques are a valuable part of hypnosis and can be especially useful during procedures that might cause discomfort, such as a dental cleaning. The main idea is to divert the patient's attention away from the sensation of the dental tools and focus it on something more pleasant and relaxing.

A common distraction technique is visualization. In this case, the dentist might guide the patient to imagine that he or she is in a quiet, relaxing environment, such as a tranquil garden, a sunny beach, or a serene forest. He or she might describe this place in detail, helping the patient to imagine the sounds, smells, and tactile sensations of this place. This mental distraction can help reduce the perception of discomfort during dental cleaning.

Another distraction technique could be the use of music or soothing sounds. The dental professional may be able to get the patient to focus on the music or sounds, helping to divert his or her attention away from the sensations of the dental tools.

In short, each patient is different and some techniques may be more effective than others. A hypnosis practitioner can work with each patient to determine which techniques are most appropriate for them and provide guidance and support throughout the process. With hypnosis, many patients can experience a more comfortable and stress-free dental cleaning.

REDUCTION OF EXCESSIVE SALIVATION

Excessive salivation, or sialorrhea, is a common problem in dentistry that can complicate certain dental treatments. Patients who experience excessive salivation often require frequent suctioning, which can disrupt workflow and make dental treatments more challenging and prolonged. Therefore, the ability to control salivation through hypnosis can be an invaluable skill for dentists. Below are some hypnosis techniques that can be useful for this purpose.

Induction and Relaxation

Induction and Relaxation: In the management of excesive salivation by hypnosis in dental practice, the initial stage is hypnotic induction, designed to bring the patient into a deep state of relaxation and increased receptivity. This state is essentially an altered state of consciousness where the patient is more open to suggestions and can modify his or her perception and response to salivation.

This induction process can involve a variety of techniques. One of the most common is pro- foundational breathing, which helps to relax the body and mind. Patients can be instructed to concentrate on their breathing, inhaling and exhaling deeply, and with each breath, to relax the body and mind.

breathing, it can be suggested to them to feel more and more relaxed.

Suggestions for relaxation and calm are another key element of this stage. The dentist can suggest that every part of your body is relaxing, from head to toe, and that you are becoming increasingly calm and relaxed.

In this state of deep relaxation, patients are more receptive to suggestions and may change their perception and response to salivation. For example, they may be more able to accept the suggestion that their salivary glands are producing less saliva, or that saliva is evaporating rapidly, which may result in an actual decrease in salivation.

Direct Suggestions

Direct suggestions: A critical component in the use of hypnosis to control excessive salivation is the use of direct suggestions. This approach relies on the ability of hypnosis to influence the body's physiological responses by modulating the individual's perceptions.

In the context of salivation management, dentists may use direct suggestions to affect patients' saliva production. The exact nature of these suggestions may vary, but they often involve imaginative descriptions of physiologic processes.

For example, a dentist may suggest that the ducts that produce and release saliva in the patient's mouth are narrowing or closing. This suggestion can be communicated in a way that encourages visualization by asking the patient to imagine these ducts as pipes.

small whose diameter is becoming increasingly smaller and smaller, and whose diameter is becoming increasingly smaller.
the flow of saliva.

Alternatively, they might suggest that the salivary glands are resting or decreasing their saliva production. For example, they might ask you to visualize the salivary glands as small factories that have decided to slow down their production.

These suggestions can be reinforced during the hypnosis with repeated affirmative statements, which increases the likelihood that the patient will accept and internalize the suggestion. Over time, these direct suggestions may result in decreased salivation, facilitating the dental treatment process.

It is important to note that the success of these techniques depends largely on the dentist's ability to induce an effective hypnotic state and his or her ability to formulate and present suggestions in a way that is acceptable to the patient. Adequate training and experience in hypnosis are therefore crucial to the successful use of these techniques.

Visualization

Visualization: Visualization plays an integral role in various hypnosis techniques, including the management of excessive salivation. Visualization has been shown to have a powerful effect on the perception of the body's physiological responses and therefore may be helpful in regulating saliva production.

The aim of these visualization exercises is for the patient to associate the visualized image with an actual decrease in saliva production. It has been suggested that this association may influence the autonomic nervous system, which in turn may regulate saliva production.

As the patient practices these visualizations and associates them with decreased salivation, control of saliva production may improve over time. This can be particularly useful during dental procedures, as less salivation can make the dentist's job easier. For example, the patient can be asked to imagine that he or she is in a very hot environment, feels thirsty and his or her mouth is becoming increasingly dry. In this way, salivation can be reduced by visualizing a fictitious scenario.

Post-Hypnotic Anchors and Suggestions

Similar to other applications of dental hypnosis, anchors can be established and post-hypnotic suggestions can be given to help patients control salivation outside the dental office setting.

Anchors are responses that are 'anchored' or linked to a specific stimulus. For example, an anchor can be established in which a certain gesture, such as squeezing the thumb and index finger together, is associated with decreased saliva production. With practice, this gesture can help to trigger the desired response even outside the dentist's office.

In addition, post-hypnotic suggestions are instructions given during hypnosis that the patient is expected to follow after the session. For example, a dentist might suggest that, after the hypnosis session, the patient will notice a decrease in saliva production, especially during dental procedures.

Ericksonian Hypnosis

Ericksonian Hypnosis differs from other hypnosis approaches in that it is more indirect and allows the patient to find his or her own solution to the problems presented. Instead of giving explicit instructions or suggestions, therapists employing Ericksonian hypnosis use metaphors, stories, and indirect language techniques to bring about changes in patients' behavior or emotions.

In the context of managing excessive salivation in dentistry, the dentist could use Ericksonian hypnosis to influence the patient's physiological responses. For example, the story could be told of a spring that gradually dries up, its waters calming down, decreasing its flow until it reaches a state of calm and stillness. This metaphor could be interpreted by the patient's subconscious as a suggestion that the salivary glands decrease their production, leading to a reduction in salivation.

This approach, moreover, may be especially useful in patients who may have resistances to the idea of the hypothesis or who may be critical of more straightforward suggestions. Because metaphors and suggestions are more subtle and less directive, they may be more readily accepted by the patient's subconscious.

Each of these techniques offers a different way to address excessive salivation. By implementing these strategies in their practice, dentists can help their patients better manage this aspect of their oral health and make their dental office experiences more comfortable and less stressful. Dental hypnosis training can certainly be a valuable addition to any dentist's toolbox.

In the next chapter, we will explain in detail the training and skills needed to implement hypnosis in dental practice.

FITTING OF DENTAL APPLIANCES SUCH AS DENTURES, ORTHODONTICS, BRACES, RETAINERS, AND OTHERS

Hypnosis can be a useful tool to help patients adjust more easily to appliances such as dentures, orthodontic appliances, retainers and others. Many individuals may experience discomfort, stress or anxiety when a new dental appliance is fitted. Hypnosis can help manage these feelings and facilitate the adjustment process in the following ways:

Pain and Discomfort Management

When using hypnosis to manage the pain and discomfort associated with dental appliances, there are several techniques that can be effective. These techniques focus on changing the patient's perception of pain by using the mind to control physical sensations. Some of these techniques are described below.

Hypnotic anesthesia: This technique involves suggesting to the patient that he/she experience a decrease in sensation in the area where the pain is located. This can be accomplished by suggesting that the area is becoming "numb", "numb" or "cold". By repeating these suggestions, the patient may begin to experience an actual decrease in pain.

Time Distortion: Sometimes, the perception of time may be more intense simply because it seems that persists over a long period of time. In these cases, time distortion can be an effective technique. This involves suggesting to the patient that time is passing faster or slower. If time seems to be passing faster, the pain may seem less long-lasting.

Dissociation: This technique involves helping the patient "disconnect" from the pain sensation. This may involve visualizing that the pain is a separate object that can be removed or even suggesting that the part of the body that is experiencing the pain is separate from the rest of the body.

Sensation substitution: This technique involves replacing the sensation of pain with a more pleasant sensation. This may involve visualizing a pleasant sensation, such as warmth or coolness, and then suggesting that this sensation is replacing the painful sensation.

Stress and Anxiety Reduction

Hypnosis is a powerful tool for relieving stress and anxiety, two factors that can complicate the experience of a patient who needs to wear braces. Here are some of the approaches that can be applied in these cases:

Progressive relaxation techniques: This technique involves guiding the patient to gradually relax different parts of his or her body, usually starting with the feet and moving up to the head. During this process, the individual may be asked to imagine him/herself in a calm and peaceful place. Not only can this technique help reduce stress and anxiety, but it can also improve their perception of their body, which can be beneficial in managing any discomfort caused by the dental appliance.

Visualization: Visualization is another useful technique to re- duce stress and anxiety. In this context, the patient can be asked to imagine themselves in a scenario where they feel comfortable and confident with their dental appliance. This could involve visualizing themselves talking, eating or smiling confidently with their appliance. By repeatedly visualizing these scenarios, they may begin to feel more comfortable with the idea of wearing a dental appliance.

Calm and relaxation suggestions: During hypnosis, the therapist can give calm and relaxation suggestions. These suggestions can help change the body's response to stress and anxiety, promoting a sense of calm and well-being. For example, the dentist might suggest that each deep breath the patient takes makes him or her feel more relaxed and calm.

Self-hypnosis techniques: Patients can also learn self-hypnosis techniques that they can use on their own when feeling stressed or anxious. These techniques may include deep breathing, visualization, and the use of calming words or phrases (mantras).

Promoting Acceptance of the Dental Appliance

Accepting the use of a dental appliance is a crucial aspect of the path to improved oral health. For some patients, this step can be challenging, as it can involve a variety of emotions, including discomfort, embarrassment or even denial. In these cases, hypnosis can be a valuable tool to facilitate dental appliance acceptance.

Suggestion therapy is a technique commonly used in hypnosis, in which the dental professional provides positive suggestions to influence the patient's thinking, perception and behavior. In the context of the acceptance of the dental appliance, these suggestions may be aimed at improving the patient's perception of the dental appliance.

One way to do this is to associate the dental appliance with positive benefits. For example, the dentist might suggest that the dental appliance is a useful tool that is working to improve the patient's dental health and esthetics. They can focus these suggestions on the desired end results, such as a healthier, more attractive smile or an improved bite that makes eating easier.

In addition, you can work with the patient to change their perspective of the dental appliance, helping them to see it as a temporary and necessary step in their journey toward improving their oral health. This could involve visualizing the day when they no longer need the appliance and how their teeth will feel and look.

Finally, suggestion therapy can be used to help the patient manage any negative feelings associated with the dental appliance. For example, if he or she feels shame, the dentist can give suggestions that help the patient see that wearing a dental appliance is something to be proud of, as it demonstrates his or her commitment to his or her oral health.

Improving Dental Care Habits

Proper care of a dental appliance is vital to its effectiveness and to maintaining optimal oral hygiene. However, it can be challenging for patients to adopt and maintain these new care habits. Hypnosis can be an effective method to encourage these healthy behaviors.

Through hypnotic suggestion, you can encourage the patient to visualize the positive consequences of taking proper care of his or her appliance, such as more efficient treatment and a better final result. Similarly, you can also highlight the negative consequences of not taking proper care of their appliance, such as longer treatment or oral health problems.

An example of this might be to guide the patient through a visualization in which they imagine themselves carefully cleaning their appliance, feeling satisfied and proud of their diligence and responsibility. At the end of the cleaning, they can visualize themselves looking in the mirror and admiring their clean and shiny appliance, and feel the relief and gratification of knowing that they are taking good care of their oral health.

Post-hypnotic suggestions may also be useful in this context. For example, the dentist might suggest that every time the patient sees their toothbrush, they will feel prompted to clean their dental appliance. Or that at the end of each meal, they will feel the need to check their appliance and make sure it is clean.

In addition to appliance cleaning, hypnosis can be helpful in motivating the patient to keep appointments with the orthodontist. It could be suggested that each time they mark an appointment on their calendar or receive a reminder, they feel a sense of commitment and anticipation, reinforcing the importance of these visits.

Finally, hypnosis can be useful in helping the patient to avoid foods that might damage his or her apparatus. Through hypnotic suggestions, these foods may begin to seem less palatable, while safe and healthy foods seem more attractive.

Sensitivity and Pressure Management

Managing the sensitivity and pressure associated with the placement of a new dental appliance is one of the most effective clinical uses of hypnosis in dentistry. This discomfort, although expected in the treatment process, can cause distress in patients, especially if the sensations intensify or persist over a period of time. In this context, hypnosis can provide a valuable tool to change the subjective interpretation of these sensations, which can alleviate discomfort and improve the patient's overall experience with their dental appliance.

A commonly used approach in this regard is the "hypnotic anesthesia" technique. This technique involves inducing a hypnotic state and suggesting that the affected area (in this case, the mouth or teeth) is numb or insensitive. This may reduce or eliminate the perception of sensitivity and pressure associated with the dental appliance.

In addition to hypnotic anesthesia, reframing and reassociation techniques can be used. In reframing, uncomfortable sensations are reinterpreted as positive signs that the dental appliance is working and contributing to improving the patient's dental health and esthetics. With re-association, uncomfortable sensations can be linked to pleasant or neutralizing sensations. For example, the dentist may suggest that each time the patient feels pressure, that sensation is transformed into one of comfort or relief.

Hypnotic Progressions

Hypnotic progressions, also known as futurization or future visualization techniques, are a hypnotherapy strategy in which the subject is guided to envision a desired future. In a hypnotic state, the patient can imagine in great detail what a future experience would be like and how he or she would feel, which can help change his or her behavior or reaction in the present.

During a hypnotic progression, the oral health professional guides the patient through a future scenario, allowing the patient to experience the event as if it is already occurring. This technique is often used to help patients visualize how they will overcome challenges, achieve goals, or experience success in the future.

Preparation: Prior to appliance insertion, the specialist can guide the patient through a hypnotic process to help them anticipate and prepare for the experience. This could involve visualizing the fitting process, from the first moment of placing the appliance in the mouth to the final comfort once the appliance has settled.

Managing initial discomfort: Hypnosis can be used to help patients manage the initial discomfort that is often experienced after a new dental appliance is placed. Through a hypnotic progression, it can be suggested to the patient that the initial discomfort will diminish over time and that they will eventually become comfortable with their new appliance.

Adjustment to function: Dental appliances can affect the way a patient speaks and eats. Here, hypno- sis can be useful in helping the patient anticipate these changes and adjust to them. Hypnotic progression can include visualizing how the patient will adapt to these new sensations and how they will successfully handle any challenges that may arise.

Promoting adherence to treatment: Hypnosis can be used to promote adherence to dental appliance care and maintenance instructions. Through hypnotic progressions, the importance of following the dentist's instructions can be instilled in the patient, from cleaning the appliance to its correct use and keeping follow-up appointments.

DENTAL HYPNOSIS PEDIATRIC

Pediatric Hypnosis in Dentistry is a specialized field that uses hypnosis techniques to help children manage the fear, anxiety and pain associated with dental procedures. This approach is particularly useful for children who are afraid of the dentist or who have difficulty holding still during dental work.

During hypnosis, the dentist may introduce images and suggestions that help the child feel more relaxed and less anxious. These suggestions may also help the child better manage pain or discomfort associated with certain dental procedures.

For example, the dentist may guide the child to imagine that he or she is in a quiet, relaxing place, such as a beach or meadow. He or she may also suggest that your child feel light and comfortable, as if floating on a cloud. These images and sensations can help him or her enter a state of deep relaxation, which can make the dental procedure easier.

In addition to its use during dental procedures, hypnosis can also be useful after treatment to help children manage postoperative anxiety and pain. The dentist can use post-hypnotic suggestion to help you anticipate a calm and pain-free recovery.

It is important to note that pediatric hypnosis in dentistry is a tool that should be used as part of a comprehensive approach to pain and anxiety management. This includes appropriate anesthesia, postoperative pain relief, and emotional support for the child.

How is Hypnosis Used in Pediatric Dentistry?

In pediatric dentistry, hypnosis can be used to help children overcome the fear and anxiety associated with dental procedures. This may include creating a calm and safe environment, inducing a state of relaxation, and suggesting pleasant and positive feelings.

Relaxation Induction

Relaxation induction in pediatric dentistry through the use of hypnosis techniques is a valuable practice that can help alleviate a child's fear and anxiety. This can be accomplished through a variety of methods:

One of the most common methods is guided breathing. Dentists can guide children through a deep, controlled breathing pattern, which helps them focus on their breathing and allows them to release any tension. An example of this would be to ask him or her to imagine that your body is a balloon that inflates and deflates with each breath, promoting a greater sense of relaxation.

Another technique is guided visualization. Here, dentists may ask the child to imagine himself in a place or situation that is calming or pleasurable, such as lying on a warm beach or by a quiet stream. This focus on positive thoughts may help him or her feel more relaxed.

Progressive muscle relaxation is another useful strategy that dentists can use. In this technique, the dentist guides the child to tense and then relax each muscle group, starting from the feet and working up to the head. By doing this, the child becomes more aware of the physical sensations of relaxation, which can help relieve tension and anxiety.

Finally, the use of self-affirmations can also be helpful. These are positive statements that the child can repeat during the dental procedure to encourage positive thinking and relaxation. Examples of self-affirmations might be "I am confident and relaxed" or "Each res- piration relaxes me more and more."

Redirection of Focus of Attention

The technique of redirection of attention, through hypnosis, is a powerful practice in pediatric dentistry for managing pain and anxiety. This is accomplished by directing the child's attention away from pain and toward more pleasant experiences.

One of the ways to do this is through a sensory approach. Dentists can guide the child to focus on other, more pleasurable sensations. For example, they might suggest that the child feel how the dental chair feels.

The child may also be encouraged to hug his or her back, providing comfort and security, or to pay attention to the soothing sound of background music.

Another technique involves diverting the child's attention to pleasant thoughts. Dentists may suggest that the child imagine being in a favorite place or enjoying a favorite food. This might translate into something like, "Imagine you are in a park playing with your friends" or "Visualize you are eating your favorite dessert and taste it in your mouth."

Guided visualization can also be used to redirect the child's attention. In this technique, dentists might ask the child to imagine himself or herself in a peaceful and pleasant environment, such as a quiet meadow or a forest full of natural beauty.

The aim of these techniques is to change the child's focus of attention. Instead of focusing on pain, the child concentrates on more pleasant and soothing experiences, sensations and images. However, it is important to keep in mind that the effectiveness of these techniques may vary from patient to patient, and depends largely on the child's willingness to participate. Therefore, it is crucial that dentists have a variety of techniques at their disposal and are willing to adapt their approach to individual needs.

Post-Hypnotic Suggestions

Post-hypnotic suggestions are an important part of the use of hypnosis in pediatric dentistry. These are instructions that are given during the hypnosis session, but are intended to have a continuing effect after the session has ended.

For example, a post-hypnotic suggestion to help children manage pain or discomfort after a dental procedure might be, "After we leave the room, every time you feel discomfort, I want you to imagine that you are blowing bubbles. Each bubble you blow carries a small part of that discomfort with you, blowing it away from your mouth and making it disappear into thin air."

It may also be helpful to suggest a physical cue that can be used to trigger relaxation, such as "When you touch your ear, you will feel relaxed and comfortable."

These suggestions can be very useful in helping children deal with any postoperative discomfort at home, and can be an effective way to give them a self-help tool to manage their own pain and anxiety.

It is important that these suggestions are safe, appropriate, and explained in a way that is clear and understandable to the child. In addition, they should be positive and empowering, and designed to foster resilience and the ability to manage pain and anxiety effectively.

The effectiveness of post-hypnotic suggestions may vary from child to child, and may depend on factors such as age, willingness to participate, and ability to understand and follow instructions. Therefore, it is always important to tailor these suggestions to the child's individual needs.

Creating a Safe Environment

Creating a safe environment is a critical strategy in pediatric dentistry, especially when using hypnosis techniques. This involves transforming the dental environment, which may seem cold and intimidating to a child, into a space that is perceived as safe, welcoming, and friendly.

One of the most commonly used techniques for this purpose is guided visualization. Through hypnosis, the dentist can guide you to imagine yourself in a safe and comfortable environment. For example, the dentist might suggest, "Imagine you are in a garden full of your favorite flowers. You can hear the sound of birds singing, and the sun warms your skin. You feel completely safe and relaxed in this garden."

This not only distracts the child from any potential physical inco- modities, but also serves to change perceptions about the dental environment. By associating the dental experience with pleasant images and sensations, the dental visit becomes a more positive experience.

In addition, it is important for dentists to establish an atmosphere of trust and respect. This includes talking to the child in a friendly and respectful manner, explaining what they are going to do in a way they can understand, and giving them the opportunity to ask questions or express concerns. This can help alleviate any anxiety or fear the child may have, and make them feel more comfortable and confident during their dental visit.

Creating a safe environment in the dental office is a crucial part of pediatric dentistry, and hypnosis can be an effective tool to accomplish this. However, it is important to remember that hypnosis must be used in a manner that is safe, ethical and respectful, and always with the consent of the child and his or her parents or guardians.

In addition to visualization, hypnosis in pediatric dentistry may also include progressive muscle relaxation techniques, for example, the dentist may say, "Imagine that every part of your body is becoming as light as a feather. Start with your toes, then work your way up your legs, your stomach, your arms, all the way down to your toes, then up your legs, your stomach, your arms, all the way up to your toes.

your head. You feel how every part of your body relaxes and you feel more and more calm and confident."

The use of soft music or nature sounds can also be helpful in creating a relaxing and safe environment. These sounds can help distract the child from any potentially intimidating noises from the dental equipment and reforce the feeling of being in a safe and pleasant place.

Finally, maintaining open and empathetic communication with the child is crucial to creating a safe environment. The dentist should explain everything that is going to be done in a way that the child can understand and should give the child the opportunity to express any concerns or fears he or she may have. It may also be helpful to allow the child to have a comforting object, such as a toy or blanket, during the dental procedure.

Efficacy of Hypnosis in Pediatric Dentistry

Hypnosis has been shown to be effective in reducing fear, anxiety and pain during dental procedures in children. By providing distraction and self-control, hypnosis allows the child to feel more at ease during their visit to the dentist.

In addition, unlike other methods of pain management, such as medications, hypnosis has no physical side effects and can be used safely in conjunction with other treatments. This makes it an attractive option for pain and anxiety management in pediatric dentistry.

However, it is important to note that the effectiveness of hypnosis may vary from one individual to another and depends largely on the child's willingness to participate in the process. In addition, using hypnosis effectively requires a level of skill and training on the part of the dentist.

Therefore, while hypnosis can be a valuable tool in pediatric dentistry, its use should be considered in the context of the individual and in consultation with a properly trained health care professional.

In addition, although hypnosis can be highly effective, it should not be forgotten that the relationship between the dentist and the child plays an essential role in the success of any treatment. A dentist who is kind, patient, and who demonstrates a genuine interest in the child's well-being can enhance the effectiveness of hypnosis techniques.

It is essential for dentists to be aware of your words and actions during treatment sessions. Positive comments and praise can improve a child's confidence and make dental visits a more pleasant experience.

It is important to keep in mind that hypnosis is not a quick fix or a panacea for all anxiety or pain problems. Although it can be an effective tool, hypnosis is only one of many techniques available to help children cope with anxiety and pain during dental visits. Other techniques may include cognitive-behavioral therapy, the use of sedatives, and the administration of local anesthesia.

Finally, although hypnosis can be a valuable technique to help children manage pain and anxiety during dental visits, it is not a substitute for regular dental care and home care. Children still need to learn the importance of regular oral hygiene, including brushing and flossing, to maintain good long-term oral health.

Preparing the Child for Hypnosis

Creating a Safe and Comfortable Environment: This is an essential first step for pediatric hypnosis in dentistry. The child must feel safe and comfortable in the dental environment. This may involve adjusting the lighting and sound in the room, providing toys or books to distract the child, and even allowing the child to bring in a comforting object such as a favorite toy or blanket. We also recommend the use of weighted blankets that provide a sense of security.

Effective and Developmentally Appropriate Communication: It is important for the dentist to communicate with the child in a way that is understandable and developmentally appropriate. This may involve using simple language, clear explanations and metaphors or analogies that the child can understand. Listening and responding to the child's questions and concerns is also essential for building trust and alleviating any fears or anxieties.

Explanation and Demonstration of Hypnosis: Before hypnosis, it is beneficial to explain to the child what hypnosis is and how it works. This can be done by a simple explanation or a brief, nonthreatening demonstration, for example, by guiding the child through a simple relaxation or visualization exercise. Familiarization with the process can help alleviate any fear or anxiety he or she may have.

Preprocedure Assessment and Preparation: The dentist should assess the child's level of anxiety and willingness to participate in hypnosis. This may involve talking with the child and, if appropriate, with his or her parents about their fears and concerns. Once the child is prepared, the dentist can begin the hypnosis procedure, ensuring that the child feels safe, comfortable, and relaxed throughout the process.

1. **Creating a Safe and Comfortable Environment**

Creating a safe and comfortable environment is an essential component in preparing the child for hypnosis. Here are some aspects to consider:

Lighting and Sound: The atmosphere of the room can greatly influence how the child perceives and responds to treatment. An overly bright or noisy environment can be stimulating and distracting. Therefore, adjusting the lighting to be soft and dim, and minimizing any background noise can help create a calm and relaxing environment.

Physical Space: Providing the child with a comfortable place to sit or lie down is essential. Furniture should be appropriately sized for the child and provide adequate physical support. If the child is going to lie down, a soft blanket or pillow can add an extra sense of security and comfort.

Room décor: Visual elements can also influence a child's sense of security and comfort. Soft colors, soothing images and familiar toys or objects can help create a welcoming environment.

Parental Presence: For some children, having a parent or caregiver present during hypnosis can provide an important sense of security and support.

Consistent Routines: Maintaining consistent and predictable routines can also help create a safe environment. This may include the way the child is greeted, the sequence of preparation procedures, and the way different parts of the treatment are introduced and explained.

2. Effective and Developmentally Appropriate Communication

Effective, developmentally appropriate communication is a crucial component in preparing the child for hypnosis. Here are some aspects to consider:

Simple Language: When interacting with the child, it is important to use language that is understandable to the child. This involves using simple words, short phrases and key concepts. For example, instead of saying "we are going to give you anesthesia," it may be more effective to say "we are going to make your mouth sleep".

Clear Explanations: Procedures and techniques should be explained in a way that the child can understand. This may involve the use of metaphors or analogies that are meaningful to the child. For example, hypnosis could be described as "playing an imaginative game".

Active Listening: It is equally crucial to listen to the child's questions and concerns and respond in a reassuring and reassuring manner. This can help alleviate any fears or anxieties they may have and can strengthen the trusting relationship between the child and the dentist.

Verification of Understanding: To ensure that the child has understood, it may be helpful to ask him or her to repeat back the information or instructions in his or her own words. This can also help identify and clarify any misunderstandings.

Nonverbal Communication: In addition to words, it is important to pay attention to the child's nonverbal communication, such as body language and facial expressions. This can provide valuable information about how the child is feeling and whether he/she understands what is being explained.

3. Explanation and Demonstration of Hypnosis

The explanation and demonstration of hypnosis are crucial steps in preparing the child for the procedure. Here are some aspects to consider:

Explanation of Hypnosis: Before starting hypnosis, it is essential to explain to the child what it is and how it works. It is important to use simple, friendly language. For example, hypnosis can be described as an "imagination game" or a "trip on a magic boat. It is also vital to make sure that the child understands that he/she will be in control at all times and that he/she can stop the hypnosis if he/she does not feel comfortable.

Demonstration of Hypnosis: Once the child has a basic understanding of hypnosis, a brief demonstration may be helpful. This could involve guiding him or her through a simple relaxation or visualization exercise. Make sure the child feels comfortable and safe during this demonstration.

Clarification of Expectations: It is important to make sure that the child knows what to expect during and after hypnosis. You should explain that hypnosis can help them feel more relaxed and better handle pain or fear.

Responding to Questions and Concerns: You should be prepared to answer any questions the child may have and alleviate any concerns. Remember, the goal is for him/her to feel safe and comfortable with hypnosis.

Child's Consent: Finally, before beginning hypnosis, it is important to obtain the child's consent. Make sure the child understands that hypnosis is voluntary and that he or she can stop at any time.

4. Pre-Procedure Evaluation and Preparation

Pre-procedure assessment and preparation are critical aspects of preparing the child for hypnosis. Here are some key points to consider:

Assessment of Anxiety Level: Prior to the procedure, it is essential to assess the child's level of anxiety. This can be done through observation, conversation, and in some cases, consultation with the parents. If the child seems particularly anxious, it may be necessary to adapt the approach or consider other anxiety management techniques.

Assessment of Readiness for Hypnosis: Not all children are good candidates for hypnosis. Some may resist or be unable to concentrate sufficiently. Therefore, it is important to assess the child's willingness to participate in hypnosis. This can be done through conversation and observation, as well as by trying some simple hypnotic techniques.

Preparation for the Procedure: Once the child has been evaluated and it has been decided that hypnosis is a viable option, it is important to prepare him or her for the procedure. This involves explaining what will happen in a way that he or she can understand, and making sure that he or she feels safe and comfortable.

Comfort and Safety: Assuring the child that he or she will be safe and comfortable during the procedure is crucial. This may involve explaining the safety measures that will be taken, such as the use of anesthesia, and reiterating that the child can stop the procedure at any time if he or she is uncomfortable.

Informed Consent: Finally, although children cannot give legal consent, it is ethical and beneficial to obtain their informed assent to hypnosis.

This involves making sure that the child understands what hypnosis involves and agrees to proceed with it.

Incorporation of Parents in the Process

Active parental involvement in the hypnosis process can be very beneficial to the child's experience. Here are some ways to involve parents:

1. Communication with Parents

Communication with parents is a crucial component in the hypnosis process with children. Here are some aspects to consider:

Hypnosis Explanation: Parents should receive a full and clear explanation of what hypnosis is, how it works, and what it can and cannot do. It should be explained that hypnosis is a tool that helps children relax and concentrate, making it easier to perform dental procedures.

Context of Use: It should be explained how hypnosis will be used in the context of your child's dental treatment. This may include information on when and how hypnosis will be introduced, and how it will be integrated with other pain and anxiety management techniques.

Opportunity to Ask Questions: Parents should have the opportunity to ask questions and discuss any pre-occupations they may have. This may involve holding one or more consultation meetings, depending on the needs and preferences of the parents.

Parental Involvement: Parents should be encouraged to actively participate in treatment preparation and follow-up. This may involve learning relaxation techniques that you can practice with your child at home, and provide support and positive reinforcement for your child's coping skills.

Informed Consent: Finally, parents must give informed consent for the use of hypnosis. This involves making sure that parents fully understand what hypnosis involves, the possible risks and benefits, and the available alternatives.

2. **Parent Training in Support Techniques**

Training parents in supportive techniques is very valuable to the success of the hypnosis process. Here are some points to keep in mind:

Relaxation Techniques: Parents can learn relaxation techniques to help their child feel more calm and relaxed. This may include progressive muscle relaxation, where different muscle groups are tensed and relaxed, or guided relaxation, where a relaxing place or situation is imagined.

Deep Breathing: Deep breathing is an effective technique that parents can teach their children. By focusing on the breathing and slowing it down, the child can help him or herself relax and reduce anxiety.

Visualization: Visualization is another technique that parents can learn to teach their children. This involves imagining an image or scene that is relaxing or calming. For example, the child might imagine floating on a cloud or lying on a sunny beach.

Support During the Session: Parents can learn ways to support their child during the hypnosis session. This may include encouraging the child, maintaining a calm environment, and reinforcing the dentist's suggestions.

Home Practice: Parents can practice these techniques with their child at home to help him or her get used to them and become more comfortable with them. This can help prepare the child for hypnosis and improve its effectiveness.

3. **Role of the Parents During the Hypnosis Session**

The role of parents during the hypnosis session can be crucial to the success of the hypnosis session. Here are some ways parents can play a supportive role:

Reassuring Presence: Simply being present in the room during hypnosis can provide a great deal of comfort for the child. The familiar presence can help relieve anxiety and provide a sense of security.

Emotional Support: Parents can play an important role in providing emotional support to their child. This may involve speaking calmly and reassuringly, giving encouragement, and providing physical comfort, such as holding the child's hand if that is appropriate and helpful.

Reinforcement of Suggestions: Parents can help reinforce the dentist's hypnotic suggestions. For example, if the dentist suggests that the child imagine him/herself in a quiet, relaxing place, parents can help build this image and make it more real for the child.

Maintaining a Calm Environment: Parents can help maintain a calm and relaxed environment during the hypnosis session. This may involve minimizing distractions, speaking in a soft tone of voice, and keeping their own stress level under control.

Participation in the Process: Depending on the child's age and preferences, it may be beneficial for parents to actively participate in the hypnosis process. For example, they could participate in breathing or visualization exercises with the child.

4. Maintaining Progress at Home

Maintaining progress at home is an important part of the hypnosis process. The techniques learned during hypnosis are not only useful during dental procedures, but can also be valuable tools for managing stress and anxiety in general. Here are some tips on how parents can help maintain progress at home:

Regular Practice: The relaxation and visualization techniques learned during hypnosis can be practiced regularly at home. This can help reinforce these skills and make the child feel more comfortable using them.

Reinforcement of Positive Suggestions: Parents can help reinforce positive suggestions given during hypnosis. For example, if it was suggested during the hypnosis session that the child is brave and capable, parents can reinforce this idea at home.

Calm and Supportive Environment: Providing a calm and supportive environment at home can be very beneficial to the child. This may involve making sure that the child has a quiet place to relax and practice his or her hypnosis techniques.

Ongoing Support: Parents should be available to talk with their child about their experiences with hypnosis and to support them in their continued use of the techniques.

learned. This may involve setting up a regular time to practice together or simply being available to talk when the child needs it.

Coordination with the Dentist: It is helpful for parents to maintain open communication with the dentist to report any changes or progress they observe at home. This may allow the dentist to adjust future hypnosis sessions to maximize their effectiveness.

SPECIFIC BENEFITS OF HYPNOSIS IN CHILDREN

Improved Cooperation and Understanding

Hypnosis can be a very useful tool in pediatric dentistry to improve children's cooperation and understanding. Here are some ways in which this can work:

A. STORYTELLING

Storytelling is a powerful technique that dentists can use to make dental procedures more accessible and less intimidating. Children are often naturally inclined to imagination and storytelling, so this technique can be very effective. To achieve this, consideration should be given to the introduction of the character, the development of the story, the corresponding explanation of the procedures and finally the conclusion of the story.

A more detailed guide with examples is provided below:

Introducing the Characters: The dentist could begin by introducing the characters in the story. For example, they could introduce the dental tools as "superheroes" who are tasked with keeping teeth strong and healthy and fighting "villains" such as plaque and decay. The introduction of the characters is a fundamental step in storytelling, especially when it comes to helping them understand and cope with visits to the dentist. In order to explain more concretely, it could be explained in this way:

1. *Superheroes - the dental tools:* Each dental tool can be presented as a "superhero" with a special ability or power. For example, the toothbrush could be "Captain Cleanliness," whose superpower is to brush and scrub teeth to eliminate villains. The dental floss could be "Super Accurate," who can get into tight places where "Captain Cleanup" cannot.

2. *Villains - plaque and cavities:* The villains of history are plaque and cavities. These can be pre-sented as little monsters or bugs that try to damage teeth. For example, "Plaque Pirate" is a sticky villain that sticks to teeth and "Cavity Monster" is a bug that makes holes in teeth.

3. *Mission:* The mission of the superheroes is to keep the child's teeth healthy and strong by fighting against the villains. This mission is carried out during the visit to the dentist and also at home when the child brushes and flosses.

4. *Reinforcement of the child's role:* The child can be included in the story as a superhero as well, his "superpower" is the ability to summon superheroes (brushing and flossing his teeth) every day to fight villains.

History Development

Developing the story as the dental procedure progresses can be an excellent way to keep the child engaged and distracted. Here's how the dentist might do it:

Beginning of the story: At the beginning of the procedure, the dentist can describe how the superheroes (dental tools) are beginning their mission to protect the city (the child's teeth) from the villains (plaque and decay).

Detailed description: During the procedure, the den- tist can describe in detail what each superhero is doing. For example, they could explain how "Captain Cleanup" (the toothbrush) is scrubbing and brushing, while "String Savior" (the flosser) is reaching into the hard-to-reach places to make sure no villains are coming.

Regular updates: As the procedure progresses, the dentist can provide regular updates on how the mission is going. This can help keep the child interested in the story and distracted from any discomfort.

Incorporation of obstacles and solutions: To make the story more interesting, the dentist can also include some obstacles that the superheroes have to overcome, and how they find solutions to these problems. For example, they could describe how "Captain Cleanup" has trouble getting to a particular place and how the "Savior of Corpses" comes to the rescue.

Explanation of Procedures

Through the story, the dentist can explain what is happening during the procedure in a way that the child can understand.

Here is one way in which this could be done:

Teeth cleaning: When the dentist is cleaning your teeth, you might describe how "Captain Clean" (the "Captain Clean") is used to clean your teeth.

brush) is flying around the "city" (the mouth), cleaning every "building" (tooth) he encounters. "Captain Cleanliness" uses his superpower to remove the "villanos" (plaque and cavities), leaving the city sparkling clean.

Dental exam: During the dental exam, the dentist could explain that they are using their 'Super Vision' (the dental mirror) to search for any villains that may be hiding. This could be described as an important reconnaissance mission to make sure that all villains have been eliminated.

Dental Treatments: If a den- tal treatment is needed, such as a filling, the dentist might describe it as an important repair mission. "Dr. Repairman" (the dentist) works carefully to repair any "building" (tooth) damaged by the villains.

Conclusion of the Story

At the end of the procedure, the dentist could conclude the story by telling how the "superheroes" have succeeded in their mission and left the child's teeth clean and healthy. This could help reinforce a positive association with dental procedures.

Here we present how the dentist could do it:

Celebration of success: At the end of the procedure, the den- tist could narrate how the superheroes have achieved their mi- sion. They could describe how "Captain Cleanup and String Savior" have worked together to clean up the city (the mouth) and eliminate all the villains (plaque and cavities).

Reinforcement of the results: The dentist could show the child the results of the mission, e.g., by showing the child his or her clean teeth in a mirror and explaining how look brighter and healthier thanks to the work of superheroes.

Support for the future: The dentist could reinforce that the superheroes will need the child's help to keep the city clean. This could include reminding the child about the importance of brushing and flossing every day.

Farewell to the characters: Finally, the dentist could narrate how the superheroes return to their base, ready for the next mission. This provides closure to the story and a smooth transition to the end of the visit to the dentist.

B. IMAGINATION GUIDED

Guided imagery is a relaxation technique that uses a child's imagination to promote a sense of calm and security. In the context of dentistry, it can be an effective way to help children manage the anxiety or fear they may associate with dental procedures (American Academy of Pediatrics, 2019). Here's how this technique could be used:

Creation of the Scenario

This is the first step in the guided imagination technique. It consists of asking the child to imagine a place that makes him feel happy and safe. This place can be real, such as their room or a local park, or it can be a fantasy place, such as a magical castle or a pirate island. The choice of location should be the child's to ensure that he/she feels comfortable and relaxed.

The dentist can guide you through this visualization by asking you to describe your happy place in detail. This can include the colors they see, the sounds they hear and how they feel when they are there. This process allows the child to immerse themselves in their imagination, helping to distract them from the dental procedure.

Throughout the procedure, the dentist can make references to this place, helping to keep the child in a relaxed and positive state. For example, if the child chose a pirate island as their happy place, the dentist can describe the procedure as a "treasure hunt mission" in which they are looking for "shiny gems" (clean, healthy teeth).

At the end of the procedure, the dentist can reinforce the positive experience by concluding the "treasure hunt" story, assuring the child that they have found the "treasure" (i.e., they have successfully completed the dental procedure) and can now return to their pirate island.

Guided imagery, and in particular the creation of a scenario, can be an effective tool to help children manage anxiety or fear during dental visits. By allowing the child to immerse themselves in their happy place, the dentist can help divert the child's attention away from the dental procedure and create a more pleasant experience.

Development of Details

The development of detail is a crucial aspect of guided imagery. By asking the child to describe his or her happy place in more detail, the dentist can help the child dive deeper into his or her imagination, which can provide a more effective distraction during the dental procedure.

Here are some ways your dentist might guide you in developing the details of your happy place:

Visualization: The dentist might begin by asking the child what colors he or she sees in his or her happy place. This could include the color of the sky, plants, buildings or whatever else is present in the scene.

Sounds: Next, the dentist might ask the child what sounds he or she can hear. This could include the sound of waves if the child is imagining a beach, the sound of birds if the child is imagining a forest, or any other sounds that may be present in the child's happy place.

Smells: The dentist may also ask the child what smells he or she can smell. This may help make the experience even more vivid for the child.

Touch: Finally, the dentist might ask the child to describe how things feel in his or her happy place. This might include the feel of the sand between their toes on a beach, the feel of the grass under their feet in a field, or the feel of the breeze on their face.

By asking the child to develop the details of his or her happy place, the dentist can help create a complete sensory experience. This can make the child's happy place seem more real and, therefore, more reassuring during the dental procedure. At the same time, the process of imagining and describing these details can provide an effective distraction from the dental procedure.

Transition to Dental Procedure

The transition to the dental procedure is a crucial step in the use of guided imagery in pediatric dentistry. Once the child has established and detailed

The practitioner can begin the procedure, assuring the child that he or she is in his or her safe place while dental treatment is being performed.

At this stage, the dentist can use metaphors or analogies related to the child's happy place to describe the dental procedure. For example, if the child has selected a pirate island as his or her happy place, the dentist can present the procedure as a "treasure hunt adventure" in search of "precious pearls" (clean, healthy teeth).

The dentist can remind the child during the procedure that he or she is safe and secure in his or her happy place. This constant reassurance can help keep the child calm and reduce any anxiety that may arise. In addition, the promise that the child can "return" to his or her happy place at any time can provide a sense of control and security, which can be especially helpful if the child begins to feel uncomfortable.

It is essential that the dentist maintain open and calm communication throughout the procedure, answering any questions the child may have and adapting his or her approach as needed. The ultimate goal is to ensure that the child's dental experience is as positive and stress-free as possible, and the smooth transition to the dental procedure using the guided imagery technique can be an effective tool to achieve this.

Reinforcement of Calmness and Cooperation

Reinforcing calmness and cooperation is an essential strategy during dental procedures in children. This is achieved by reminding the child of his or her "happy place" and reaffirming his or her safety and relaxation in that imaginary space.

during the dental procedure.

As the dentist proceeds with treatment, it is helpful to make regular references to the child's happy place. This may include verbal reminders that they are in their happy place, descriptions of their "dental superhero" activities there, or even questions about additional details of the happy place that the child may want to explore.

These reminders serve as effective distractions, diverting the child's attention from the procedure itself and helping him or her focus on his or her ima- gined positive experience. In addition, constant reassurance of their safety and comfort in the happy place can reinforce the child's sense of calm, helping to maintain their cooperation throughout the procedure.

It is important for the dentist to adopt a calm and soothing tone of voice during these interactions and to patiently respond to any concerns or questions the child may have. Careful and considerate management of communication during the procedure can not only contribute to the child's calmness and cooperation, but can also help build a trusting relationship between the child and the dentist, facilitating future visits to the dentist.

C. SUGGESTIONS POSITIVE

Positive suggestions are one of the most valuable tools of hypnosis, especially when it comes to working with children. In the context of pediatric dentistry, these suggestions can help children form positive associations with dental care and feel more comfortable and cooperative during procedures (Ame- rican Society of Clinical Hypnosis, 2021). Here are some examples of how they might be used:

Courage Reinforcement

Reinforcement of courage is an important tactic that dentists can employ during dental procedures in children. This strategy involves praising the child's bravery and ability to handle the dental procedure with courage.

Dentists can begin this reinforcement by encouraging the child before the procedure, reassuring him or her that he or she has the courage to handle the situation. During the procedure, the dentist can continue to reaffirm the child's bravery. For example, they may make comments such as "You are doing a great job being so brave" or "I am very impressed with how brave you are being."

Reinforcement of bravery serves to increase the child's confidence in his or her ability to handle the situation. This can help reduce anxiety and increase cooperation during the procedure. At the same time, praise and re- cognition of the child's bravery can help to promote a positive self-image and encourage resilience in future situations that may provoke anxiety.

It is important for the dentist to be genuine and sincere in his or her praise. Children are good detectors of sincerity, and genuine praise can have a significant effect on their disposition and confidence.

Therefore, reinforcement of bravery is a valuable strategy that can enhance children's dental experience, increasing their confidence and cooperation and decreasing their anxiety. This approach can turn what might be a dreaded process into an empowering experience for the child.

Association of Procedures with Pleasant Experiences

Associating procedures with pleasant experiences is an effective technique used in pediatric dentistry to create a positive experience for the child. This technique involves associating aspects of the dental procedure with experiences that the child finds pleasant or comforting.

For example, the dentist may suggest that the dental chair is like a "soft, comfortable cloud." This simple association can transform the child's perception of the dental chair from a clinical object to something familiar and pleasant.

The dentist can also use guided imagination to associate dental instruments and procedures with pleasant experiences. For example, he or she may describe the electric toothbrush as a "tickle brush" that makes the teeth laugh, or may describe the mouthwash as a "bubble bath" for the teeth.

These associations can help to demystify the dental process and make the child feel more at ease during the procedure. By associating the dental procedure with pleasant experiences, the dentist can help reduce the child's anxiety and foster a positive attitude toward dental care.

It is important that these associations are appropriate for the child's age and preferences, and that the dentist is sensitive to the child's reactions and adjusts his or her approach as needed. With the right approach, associating procedures with pleasant experiences can be a valuable tool for enhancing the dental experience for children.

Promotion of Cooperation

Encouraging cooperation is an essential aspect of pediatric dentistry. Dentists can use a variety of strategies to encourage cooperation during dental procedures, such as explaining the importance of strong, healthy teeth in a simple and understandable way.

To begin, the dentist could inform the child about the importance of strong, healthy teeth. This could be done through stories, analogies or even educational games that are appropriate for the child's age. For example, you could compare the teeth to soldiers in a castle, explaining that just as the soldiers need to be strong and healthy to protect the castle, the teeth need to be strong and healthy to protect the mouth.

Next, the dentist may explain that in order for the teeth to remain strong and healthy, they need your child's help during the dental procedure. This might involve cooperating by opening his or her mouth when asked, or holding still while the dentist examines his or her teeth.

teeth. The idea that the child's cooperation is essential for the success of the procedure can be reinforced.

Finally, you could reinforce the child's cooperation by praising him or her for his or her behavior during the procedure. This can serve as positive reinforcement that encourages the child to continue to cooperate on future dental visits.

By encouraging cooperation in this way, the dentist can help create a positive dental experience for the child, which can lead to better long-term oral health outcomes.

Calmness Promotion

Promoting calmness during dental procedures is a fundamental approach in pediatric dentistry. Dentists can use a variety of techniques to help alleviate anxiety and promote a relaxed state in the child.

A common strategy is the use of guided imagery, which has already been discussed in detail. With guided imagery, the dentist can help the child visualize a happy and safe place. This place, filled with pleasant images and sensations, can serve as an effective distraction and promote a state of calm.

In addition, you can use breathing and relaxation techniques. For example, before and during the dental procedure, the dentist could guide the child through deep breathing exercises, which can help reduce anxiety and promote relaxation.

Another strategy is effective and reassuring communication. The dentist can explain the procedure in a friendly and understandable manner, reassuring the child that he or she will be by your child's side throughout the entire process. By maintaining a calm and reassuring tone of voice, the dentist can help alleviate any fear or nervousness the child may feel.

Promoting calmness is an essential aspect of the child's dental experience. By fostering a calm and relaxed environment, you can help the child better manage the dental procedure and reduce any anxiety associated with dental care.

Pride Stimulus

Encouraging pride is an effective tactic that dentists can employ to encourage cooperation during dental procedures in children. By emphasizing that cooperation and courage during the procedure is something the child can be proud of, a positive and cooperative attitude can be encouraged.

Before the procedure, the dentist can explain to the child that cooperating during dental treatment is an act of courage and responsibility. They can emphasize that caring for teeth is an important task and that by cooperating during the procedure, the child is taking active steps to keep his or her teeth strong and healthy.

During the procedure, the dentist can reinforce this message by praising the child for his or her bravery and cooperation. They might make comments such as "You are doing a fantastic job of cooperating" or "You must feel very proud of how brave you are being".

These comments can help the child associate cooperation during dental procedures with a sense of pride and accomplishment. This may not only encourage cooperation in the moment, but may also help the child to to foster a positive attitude toward dental care in the future.

It is important for the dentist to be authentic in his or her elo gations and comments, as children are sensitive to sincerity. In doing so, the strategy of stimulating pride can be an effective tool to encourage cooperation and enhance the dental experience in children.

D. RELAXATION TRAINING

Relaxation training is a valuable tool that can be taught to children during hypnosis sessions to help them manage stress or anxiety associated with dental procedures. Common relaxation techniques include deep breathing, progressive muscle relaxation, and visualization (American Society of Clinical Hypnosis, 2021). Here's how children might be taught these techniques:

Deep Breathing

Deep breathing is, in fact, an extremely effective relaxation technique that is often used in stressful or anxious situations, and is especially useful in a pediatric dental setting. This technique is based on the principle that conscious control of breathing can have a calming effect on the nervous system, helping to reduce anxiety and promote relaxation.

To teach the child the deep breathing technique, the dentist can start by explaining in a simple and friendly way what they are going to do. They can tell the child that they are going to do a "breathing game" that will help the child feel more comfortable and relaxed.

You can then guide the child through the steps of deep breathing. You can instruct the child to inhale slowly for a count of three, hold the breath for a moment, and then exhale slowly for another count of three. The dentist can demonstrate this first so the child can see exactly what to do.

While the child practices deep breathing, the dentist can offer words of encouragement and praise, reinforcing the positive behavior. By focusing on breathing, the child can be distracted from any discomfort or anxiety, which can facilitate a calmer and more positive dental experience.

It is important for the dentist to be patient and encouraging during this process, as it may take some time for the child to become comfortable with the deep breathing technique. However, with practice and proper guidance, this technique can be a valuable tool in helping children manage dental anxiety.

Progressive Muscle Relaxation

Progressive muscle relaxation is a stress and anxiety management technique that can be particularly useful in a dental setting. By intentionally tensing and relaxing different muscle groups, children can develop a greater awareness of physical sensations of stress and learn to counteract them.

To guide a child through progressive muscle relaxation, the dentist can begin by explaining the technique in a simple and friendly way. They might describe it as a "flexion and relaxation game" that will help make the child feel more comfortable.

The dentist can then guide the child through the process of tensing and relaxing the different muscle groups. Typically, you start with the muscles in the feet and work your way up to the muscles in the head. For example, you might say, "Now, imagine that you are squeezing all the muscles in your feet, as if you were trying to grasp a pencil with your toes. Hold that tension... and now relax."

It is important that the dentist go at a pace that is comfortable for the child and provide plenty of praise and positive reinforcement along the way. By the end of the sequence, the child may have developed a greater sense of relaxation and calmness.

Progressive muscle relaxation can be a valuable tool to help children manage anxiety in the dental office. However, as with any new skill, it may take some practice for the child to become comfortable with the technique.

Visualization

Visualization or guided imagery is a powerful technique that can help children manage anxiety and achieve a state of deep relaxation. This technique involves guiding the child to visualize an image or scene that is soothing and pleasing to him or her.

For example, the dentist may ask the child to close his or her eyes and imagine that he or she is in a place that he or she likes very much, such as a sunny beach, a meadow full of flowers, or floating on a soft cloud. The dentist can help make the image more vivid by describing the details of the scene, such as the feel of the warm sand underfoot on the beach or the softness of the cloud.

Visualization can be used in conjunction with deep breathing and progressive muscle relaxation. For example, while the child is breathing deeply and relaxing his muscles, the dentist can suggest that each breath makes him feel more and more relaxed, as if he is floating on a soft cloud.

Visualization can be particularly useful in a dental environment, as it can help distract the child from the procedure and focus on pleasant images and sensations. This technique may take some practice, but with proper guidance, it can be an effective tool for reducing dental anxiety in children.

E. POST-HYPNOTIC SUGGESTIONS

Post-hypnotic suggestions are instructions or ideas given during a hypnosis session that the subject will carry out or remember after the session has ended. In the context of pediatric dentistry, these su- gerences can be an effective tool to help children remember their dental visit in a positive way and encourage cooperation in future visits (American Socie- ty of Clinical Hypnosis, 2021). Here's how they could be used:

Remembering the Visit in a Positive Way

Remembering the dental visit in a positive way is an effective strategy for relieving anxiety about future visits. At the end of the procedure, the dentist can discuss with the child how well he or she did and how much he or she contributed to keeping the teeth strong and healthy. This can help reinforce the idea that the dental visit was a positive experience.

It may also be helpful to provide positive reinforcement, such as praise, stickers or small toys, at the end of the visit. This may help the child associate the dental visit with positive rewards, which may motivate the child to cooperate on future visits.

By encouraging the child to remember the visit in a positive way, the dentist can help alleviate any anxiety the child may have about future visits and foster a positive attitude toward dental care.

Reinforcing Cooperative Behavior

Reinforcing cooperative behavior is a very effective strategy in pediatric dentistry. The goal is to help the child associate cooperative behaviors with positive outcomes, which in turn may motivate the child to repeat these behaviors in the future.

For example, the dentist can praise the child during and after the procedure for his or her cooperation and bravery. Phrases such as "You did a great job opening your mouth so wide" or "I am very impressed with how brave you were today" can help reinforce cooperative behavior."

Finally, it is important for the dentist to communicate these successes to the child's parents or caregivers so that they can continue to reinforce these positive behaviors at home. By working together, the dentist and parents can help foster a positive and cooperative attitude toward dental visits.

Promoting Good Oral Hygiene Habits

Promoting good oral hygiene habits is an essential aspect of pediatric dentistry. The goal is to help the child understand the importance of daily oral care, and to develop healthy routines that will last a lifetime.

During the visit, the dentist can talk to the child about the importance of brushing and flossing every day. You can explain in a simple, friendly way how these habits help keep teeth strong and healthy and prevent dental problems.

In addition, the dentist can demonstrate proper brushing and flossing techniques and allow the child to practice in the office. This can help the child feel more comfortable and confident with these practices at home.

It can also provide positive reinforcement to motivate the child to maintain good oral hygiene habits.

Finally, it is important for the dentist to communicate with the child's parents or caregivers so that they can continue to reinforce these habits at home. Through education and positive reinforcement, the dentist can help the child develop healthy oral hygiene habits that will last a lifetime.

Associating Positive Emotions with Dental Care

Associating positive emotions with dental care can be an effective strategy for encouraging good oral hygiene habits in children. Rather than viewing dental care as a chore or an obligation, the goal is to help the child see it as a way to take care of themselves and take pride in their health.

The dentist can help foster these positive associations in a number of ways. For example, they can praise the child for his or her effort and dedication to brushing and flossing, reinforcing the idea that these are behaviors of which they can be proud.

In addition, they can talk about the satisfaction and confidence that comes with having clean, healthy teeth. For example, they can say things like "You must feel very good knowing that you are taking good care of your teeth" or "Having clean, healthy teeth is something you can be very proud of".

In summary, by associating positive emotions with dental care, the dentist can help motivate the child to maintain good oral hygiene habits and cultivate a positive attitude toward dental health that will last a lifetime.

REDUCTION OF ANXIETY AND FEAR

Hypnosis can be an effective tool for reducing the anxiety and fear that children often feel in relation to dental visits. Children may experience fear and anxiety related to dental procedures due to a variety of factors, such as pain, discomfort, noise, and fear of the unknown. Hypnosis can help children manage these feelings, which can make dental visits less stressful and more comfortable. Here's how some of these techniques might be used:

RELAXATION TECHNIQUES

Relaxation techniques can be extremely helpful in situations that cause stress or anxiety, such as a visit to the dentist. Here is how these techniques could be implemented:

Deep Breathing

Deep breathing, such as "square breathing," is an excellent relaxation technique that can be very beneficial for both children and adults.

To implement it in a dental office, the dentist could guide the child through the process step by step. They could start by explaining what square breathing is in a simple and friendly way, and then demonstrate how to do it.

The dentist could then guide the child through the technique: inhale for four seconds, hold the breath for four seconds, exhale for four seconds, and then hold the lungs empty for four seconds. This cycle would be repeated several times.

During the process, you can remind the child to focus on breathing, helping to distract the child from any anxiety or discomfort he or she may be feeling. You can also praise the child for his or her effort, reinforcing positive behavior.

Square breathing can be particularly helpful during dental procedures that may cause anxiety, as it can help calm the nervous system and reduce stress. However, as with any new ha- bility, it can take some time for the child to feel comfortable with the technique. With patience and practice, it can become a valuable tool for managing dental anxiety.

After deep breathing, other relaxation techniques can be implemented.

Progressive Muscle Relaxation

Progressive muscle relaxation is an effective technique for reducing anxiety and promoting relaxation. Here I provide you with a detailed description of how this technique could be implemented in a dental setting for children:

Initial explanation: The dentist might begin by explaining the technique to the child in a way that is easy to understand. He or she might say something like, "We are going to play a tension and relaxation game. In this game, we are going to learn to tense and relax different parts of our body, starting with our toes and working our way up to our heads.

Feet and legs: The dentist might instruct the child to tense the muscles in the feet and legs and then relax them. He or she might say something like, "Now, imagine that you are tightening the muscles in your feet as if you were trying to grasp a pencil with your toes. Hold that tension for a few seconds... and then relax.

Abdomen and chest: Then, you could guide the child through the process of tensing and relaxing the muscles of the abdomen and chest.

Arms and hands: Next, the child could learn to tense and relax the muscles of the arms and hands.

Face and head: Finally, the child may learn to hold and relax the muscles of the face and head.

It is important that the dentist go at a pace that is comfortable for the child and provide plenty of praise and positive reinforcement along the way. With practice, this technique can help the child manage anxiety and promote a greater sense of calm during dental visits.

VISUALIZATION OF RELAXATION

This technique can be used in combination with deep breathing and progressive muscle relaxation. The child might be guided to visualize a calm scene, such as a beach or meadow. This approach can help distract the child from any fear or anxiety he or she may feel.

1. DISPLAY

Visualization is a powerful technique that can help children manage their anxiety during visits to the dentist. Here's how you might implement it:

Creation of the Scenario

Creating a scenario is a crucial component of the visualization technique and can be a very effective way of diverting the child's attention away from the dental experience and toward something pleasant and reassuring.

Here is a detailed description of how a dentist might guide a child through this process:

Home

The dentist might begin by saying something like, "We're going to play an imagination game. I want you to think of a place or experience that makes you feel happy and safe.

It may be a real place you know, or it may be a fantasy place you'd like to visit."

Choice of location

The child then chooses his or her spot. The dentist might ask questions to help the child describe the spot in detail, such as "What colors do you see?" or "Are there any sounds in this spot?"

Scenario creation

Once the child has described his or her location, the practitioner can help create a more detailed scenario. For example, if the child has chosen a local park, the dentist might say, "Imagine you are in your favorite park. You can feel the fresh grass under your feet, hear the birds singing, see the green trees and the blue sky.

Maintaining the visualization

During the dental procedure, you can remind the child of his or her happy place, helping him or her to remain in a relaxed state.

This visualization technique can help reduce anxiety and discomfort during dental visits by providing the child with a positive and comforting distraction.

The dentist might begin by asking the child to imagine a place or experience that is comforting to him or her. It may be a place the child is familiar with, such as his or her bedroom or a local park, or a fantasy place, such as a magical castle or pirate island.

Development of Details

Developing details in the visualization helps make the experience more vivid and engaging for the child. Here's how a dentist might do it:

1. Beginning: The dentist might begin by encouraging the child to explore his or her chosen place or experience with all of his or her senses. She might say something like, "Let's imagine what this place is really like. Let's use all of our senses to make this place as real as possible."

2. Vision: You might ask the child about the colors he or she sees. For example, "What colors can you see around you? Is there anything that shines or catches your eye?"

3. Sound: Next, you might ask the child about sounds. For example, "What sounds can you hear - is it calm and quiet, or can you hear the sound of waves, birds singing, or perhaps other people laughing and playing?"

4. Smell: Next, you might ask the child about smells. For example, "Is there a smell in the air?
Can you smell the flowers, the sea, or maybe your food? favorite?"

5. Touch: Finally, you might ask the child about how things feel in this place. For example, "How does the ground feel under your feet-is it soft, hard, warm, or cold?"

By involving all of the child's senses in the visualization, the dentist can make the imaginary place more real and appealing, which can increase the effectiveness of the technique in reducing anxiety and promoting relaxation.

Use During the Procedure

The visualized safety place can be a great tool for the child during the dental procedure.

Here we show how a dentist might guide a child through this process:

Reminder of the safe place

The dentist can prepare the child for the dental procedure by actively reminding the child of his or her imagined safe place. This can be done by saying something like, "Think of your special place, that place where you feel safe and happy. Close your eyes and go there in your mind's eye".

As the procedure progresses, you can continue to direct the child toward that visualization. This can be done by asking questions that help keep the image alive, such as: "What are you doing in your special place now?
What colors do you see?"

If the child seems distracted or nervous at any time, you can help redirect his attention back to his safe place. This can be done by gently reminding him of the place and asking him to imagine himself there again.

At the end of the procedure, you should congratulate the child on his or her courage and remind him or her of how his or her safe place helped him or her get through the procedure. This can help reinforce the importance and effectiveness of visualization as a stress management tool.

The goal of remembering the safe place is to help the child focus on positive thoughts and feelings, rather than on the anxiety or fear that may be associated with the dental procedure. With practice, this technique can be a valuable tool for stress management in a variety of situations.

Guidance during the procedure

During the dental procedure, the dentist can guide the child to keep his or her attention on his or her imagined safe place. This guidance can be through questions or statements that make the child's visualization more vivid and realistic.

For example, at the beginning of the procedure, you could remind the child of the safe place he/she has imagined and ask him/her to imagine him/herself there.

As you go through the procedure, you can ask questions that help keep the scene vivid in the child's mind, such as, "Can you see the beautiful colors around you? Can you hear the peaceful sounds in your safe place?"

If at any time the child seems anxious, you can redirect his or her attention back to its safe place with gentle reminders and visualization-focused questions.

Once the procedure is completed, the dentist can praise the child for his or her ability to remain calm and focused in his or her safe place, thus reinforcing the value of this technique.

This method helps to divert the child's attention away from any discomfort or anxiety they may feel during the dental procedure, and instead allows them to focus on their safe place, which can help reduce anxiety and promote relaxation.

Positive reinforcement

Positive reinforcement can be a powerful tool to help children handle situations that may seem difficult or scary. Here's how a dentist might do it:

Praise during the procedure: As the child undergoes the dental procedure, the dentist can offer words of encouragement and praise. For example, he or she might say, "You are doing a fantastic job. You are very brave.

Reinforcing visualization: In addition to general praise, the dentist can specifically praise the child's commitment to the visualization technique. For example, he or she might say, "You are doing a great job visualizing yourself in your safe place. I am impressed with how well you are doing."

Reminder of achievement: At the end of the procedure, you can remind the child of how well he or she has done, both in terms of his or her behavior during the procedure and his or her use of the visualization technique. For example, the dentist might say, "You did very well today. I am very proud of how brave you were and how well you used your safe place."

Positive reinforcement can help increase a child's confidence in his or her ability to handle difficult situations and can make him or her feel more comfortable and confident during dental visits. In addition, it can reinforce the use of visualization as a useful technique for managing stress and anxiety.

Return to the safe place

Returning to the safe place is an effective strategy for the dentist to use if he or she notices that the child feels anxious or uncomfortable at any time during the procedure. Here is one way you might do this:

Observation: The dentist should watch for signs of discomfort or anxiety in the child. This may include changes in the child's behavior, body language or facial expression.

Safe place reminder: If the child begins to show signs of anxiety, the practitioner can gently remind the child to return to his or her safe place in his or her mind. For example, you might say, "Remember your safe place. Imagine you are there now. What do you see? What do you hear?"

Reinforcing visualization: You can continue to ask questions about the safe place to help the child refocus his or her attention. For example, you might say, "Are there any special sounds in your safe place? What does the air feel like there?"

Continuation of the procedure: Once the child is more relaxed and centered in his or her safe place, the dentist can continue with the procedure.

This technique can be very useful in helping the child manage anxiety during dental visits. In addition, by learning to use this technique on his or her own, the child can gain a valuable tool for managing stress in a variety of situations.

Reinforcing Calm

The dentist can use the child's place of safety as a tool to reinforce calmness and cooperation during the dental procedure. Here is one way this might work:

Constant reminder: Throughout the procedure, you can remind the child of his or her place of safety by asking about the specific details you have imagined. This can help keep the child focused and calm.

Use a calm tone: You can use a soft, soothing tone of voice when talking to the child about his or her place of safety. This can reinforce the sense of calm and safety that the child associates with his or her imagined place.

Reinforcing cooperation: You can also link the child's cooperation to his or her ability to stay in his or her safe place. For example, the dentist might say, "You do a great job staying calm and cooperating, just like you would in your safe place."

Praise for calmness: You can praise the child for being calm and cooperative, thus reinforcing positive behavior. For example, the dentist might say, "I am very impressed with how calm and cooperative you have been. You've done a great job of imagining yourself in your safe place."

The use of these strategies can help keep the child calm and cooperative during the dental procedure, which can make the experience less stressful for both the child and the dentist.

SUGGESTIONS POSITIVE

Positive suggestions can be a powerful tool for changing a child's attitude toward dental visits.

Here we show how a dentist could use positive sugerences:

Before the Procedure

This is an excellent way to prepare the child for the procedure. By framing the dental visit as an exciting opportunity to take care of their teeth, the dentist can help allay any fears or anxieties the child may have.

In addition, pre-procedure discussion may also include:

Simple explanation

Clear and simple communication is critical when presenting a child for a dental procedure. By explaining what will happen in a way the child can understand, the dentist can help alleviate any fear or anxiety the child may have about the unknown.

Here are some key elements you may want to consider when explaining the procedure:

Age-appropriate language: The dentist should be sure to use language that is appropriate for the child's age and understanding. This could include referring to dental equipment with objects or experiences familiar to the child. For example, the dental probe could be referred to as a "little spoon" that is used for "counting teeth."

Step-by-step description: Explaining each step of the procedure before it happens can help prepare the child for what is to come. For example, you might say, "First, I'm going to look at your teeth with my little spoon, then I'll clean them with a special brush, and finally I'll rinse them with water."

Focus on the positive aspects: The dentist should try to focus on the positive aspects of the procedure. For example, he or she might say, "After we clean your teeth, they will be as bright and clean as the stars in the sky.

Invitation to ask questions: You should invite the child to ask any questions he or she has. This can help the child feel more in control and alleviate any concerns he or she may have.

By explaining in a simple and friendly way what will happen during the procedure, the dentist can help ease the child's fear of the unknown and prepare him or her for a positive dental experience.

Focus on results

Indeed, focusing on positive outcomes can be a very effective way to help children understand and appreciate the value of dental visits.

1. Highlight visible results: The dentist can describe how the teeth will look after the procedure. For example, he or she might say, "At the end of our visit, your teeth will be so bright and clean that you will be able to see your reflection in them."

2. Emphasize the feeling of cleanliness: In addition to how the teeth will look, you can talk about how they will

your teeth will feel. I might say, "Your teeth will feel so smooth and clean. It will be like having a new set of teeth."

3. Associate with positive emotions: You can associate the feeling of clean teeth with positive emotions. For example, you might say, "You're going to feel great with your bright, healthy smile. I'm sure you won't be able to stop smiling."

4. Relate to overall health: Finally, you can relate clean, healthy teeth to the child's overall health. For example, you might say, "Keeping your teeth clean and healthy is a very important part of keeping your whole body healthy."

These explanations can help children understand the value of dental visits and anticipate the positive results they can expect. This can make them feel more comfortable and excited about the procedure.

Inclusion of parents

Parental involvement can be crucial in helping a child feel safe and understood during a dental visit.

Pre-procedure conversation: Before the procedure, the practitioner can talk with the parents and child together to explain what will happen. Parents can re- force what the dentist says and help alleviate any fears or concerns the child may have.

Support during the procedure: During the procedure, if possible, parents can be present in the room to offer emotional support. Your presence can be a great comfort to the child.

Involvement in the storytelling: If the dentist is using storytelling to help explain the procedure, parents can be involved in the story. For example, they could play a role in the story or help add details.

Post-procedure conversation: After the procedure, the dentist can talk with the parents and child together again. They can discuss how the procedure went, highlight the child's positive behaviors and talk about the next steps for the child's dental care.

Including the parents in the entire process can provide an additional layer of support and security for the child. This can help alleviate any anxiety the child may have and ensure that they feel comfortable and cared for during their dental visit.

The goal is to make the child feel at ease and excited about the dental visit, which can make the experience much more enjoyable and less stressful for everyone involved.

During the Procedure

Continued use of positive suggestions during the procedure can help keep the child calm and cooperative. Here we show how a dentist might do this:

Acknowledging cooperation: As the child sits in the chair and the procedure continues, the dentist may say something like, "You are doing a great job of staying calm and cooperating with me. This is really helping to keep your teeth strong and healthy."

Praise for calmness: If the child remains calm during the procedure, you can reinforce this behavior with further praise, such as, "I'm impressed with how calm you are being. That makes my job much easier, and it helps you too.

Focus on the benefits: You can repeat the benefits of the child's cooperation and calmness, such as, "By staying calm and working with me, you are helping your teeth stay clean and healthy. That's great."

These comments will help the child associate the dental visit with positive experiences and feelings, which can make future dental visits less stressful.

After the Procedure

It is crucial to reinforce the child's positive attitudes toward dental visits after the procedure. Here's how the dentist might do it:

Praise for effort: You can begin by congratulating the child for completing the procedure. You might say, "You did an amazing job today. I really appreciate your cooperation.

Reinforcing the results: You can then highlight the positive results of the procedure. You might say, "Look how clean and healthy your teeth are now. You should be very proud of yourself.

Focus on the future: Finally, you can encourage the child for future dental visits. You might say, "I look forward to seeing you again for your next checkup. If you keep taking care of your teeth the way you did today, you will always have a healthy, bright smile."

These comments help to solidify the child's positive experience and create a positive association with dental visits. This can make future visits easier and less stressful for the child.

The use of positive suggestions can help relieve the child's anxiety and promote a positive attitude toward dental visits. By focusing on the positive aspects of the dental visit, the dentist can help the child associate the dental visit with feelings of joy and excitement, rather than fear or anxiety.

STORYTELLING:

Storytelling can be an effective tool to help children understand and manage dental visits.

Create a Scenario

Creating a scenario or story is an effi- cient technique to make the environment less intimidating and more understandable to children. By using metaphors, the dentist can explain dental procedures in a way that the child can understand and accept. For example, comparing the oral cavity to a castle, the teeth to soldiers defending the castle, and the bacteria to the invaders can help children understand the importance of oral hygiene.

In addition, creating a setting that is friendly and appealing to children can distract them from the actual procedure. This may involve decorating the dental clinic with bright colors, cartoon characters or even the inclusion of games or play activities.

The use of child-friendly language and terms is also essential to put children at ease. For example, instead of saying "I'm going to extract this tooth," the practitioner might say, "Let's help this baby tooth to be removed so that a bigger, stronger tooth can take its place."

Finally, by incorporating play elements into the visit, the dentist can make the visit more fun and less frightening for children. This may include rewarding children with stickers or small toys at the end of their visit to positively reinforce their experience at the dentist.

In summary, by creating a scenario or story, the dentist can transform the dental experience from something potentially frightening to something understandable, educational and even exciting for children. This approach can contribute to a positive attitude toward dental health in general, encourage cooperation during dental visits, and encourage children to adopt good oral hygiene habits in the long run.

Here is a way to expand this concept:

Introduction

Here we present how a dentist might introduce a story:

Beginning of the story: "Did you know that your teeth are like precious diamonds in a fortress? But there are little dragons, which are the bacteria, that are trying to slice those diamonds".

Description of the problem: "These little dragons, the bacteria, love sweets as much as you do and if you don't stop, they can tarnish your diamonds, making them less bright and strong."

Introducing the hero: "But don't worry, because I'm here to help you. As your dentist, I'm like a va- liant guardian, equipped with magical tools to keep those little dragons at bay and protect your precious diamonds."

Invitation to collaboration: "But I need your courage. I need you to open your mouth wide so I can see all your diamonds and make sure they are shiny and strong. Are you ready to defend your fortress together?"

Promise of success: "If we work together, we can keep your diamonds, your teeth, shiny, strong and healthy. Are you ready to embark on this exciting mission?"

This narrative turns the visit to the dentist into a heroic adventure, helping children understand the process and feel more comfortable and engaged.

Development of the conflict

Then the dentist can continue the story, saying, "These little monsters, or bacteria, can make little holes in the towers of your castle if we don't detect them. But don't worry, because that's exactly what we're here to do."

That's right, developing the conflict can make the story more exciting and engaging for the child. Here's a way to expand this part of the story:

Description of the problem: "These little monsters, the bacteria, are very cunning. If we don't stop them, they can start making small tunnels in the towers of your castle, which can make the towers not as strong as they should be."

Aggravating the conflict: "And once the monsters have tunneled into a tower, it's easier for them to tunnel back in. That's why it's so important to stop them before they can start."

Promise of solution: "But don't worry, that's exactly what I'm here for. As your dentist, I have the tools and skills to detect these little monsters and stop them before they can do damage to your castle."

Invitation to participate: "But I need your help. I need you to be brave and open your mouth wide so I can see all the towers of your castle. Together, we can stop these monsters and keep your castle strong and healthy".

By developing conflict in this way, the dentist can help children understand the importance of dental care and feel more involved in the process. This can result in a more positive and less stressful dental visit for the child.

Presentation of the heroes

By presenting himself or herself as the hero of the story, the dentist can help alleviate any fear or anxiety the child may have.

Hero's introduction: "Just like the brave knights who protect castles in stories, I, as your dentist, am here to protect your castle. My team and

I am like a team of knights, ready to defend you from the little monsters.

Description of tools: "I have a number of special tools, each with its own magic. For example, my dental mirror is like a magic shield that allows me to see all the nooks and crannies of your castle. My dental probe is like a sword that helps me check if the monsters have been tunneling."

Guarantee of protection: "With these tools and our courage, we can make sure that all the little monsters are chased away and that your castle, your teeth, remain strong and shiny".

Invitation to join the team: "But we need your help. You have to be our brave prince or princess, ready to help us defend your castle. Are you ready to join us in this adventure?"

By presenting as the hero and making the child feel part of the team, the dentist can help make the dental experience more exciting and less intimidating for the child. This can result in a more positive and less stressful visit to the dentist.

Involve the child

By including the child as an integral character in the story, the child's active participation is encouraged and any potential anxiety is reduced. Let's look at how the dentist might con- tinue this narrative:

Turning the child into a hero: "But, even the bravest of the bravest of cowboys need help. That's why I need your bravery. You are a crucial guardian of this castle. Are you ready to take on that responsibility?"

Child's task description: "One of the most important ways you can help us is to be brave and open your mouth wide when I ask you to. This way, I will be able to see all the towers in your castle and make sure they are safe from the little monsters."

Praise for the child's courage: "I know you can do it, because you are incredibly brave. And remember, you're not in this alone. We're here to help you and together, we can keep your castle strong and shining."

Closing or End of story

Giving the child an active and vital role in the story can make the experience more positive and less frightening. Here's how the dentist might close the story:

Plan review: "So, we've talked about the little monsters, the bacteria, trying to tunnel into the towers of your castle, right? And we've talked about how we, the dental knights, are going to defend your castle."

Confirmation of the child's role: "But, most importantly, we have talked about how you are going to be a brave guardian of your own castle. You are going to help us by opening your mouth wide when necessary and being brave throughout the process."

Call to action: "So, are you ready to start our adventure? Are you ready to defend your castle and make sure it stays strong and shiny?"

Recognition of the child's courage: "I know you can do it, because you are the bravest guardian I know. Together, let's make this visit to the dentist an exciting adventure.

Detail the Procedure

Keeping the narrative going during the procedure can help keep the child engaged and distracted from any possible discomfort. Here's how the dentist might do it:

Start of the procedure: "Now that you are a brave guardian, let's begin our adventure. First, I'm going to use my magic mirror to inspect all the towers in your castle. This doesn't hurt at all, it's just so you can see everything clearly."

Cleaning: "Now I'm going to use my magic brush to smoke out the bacteria monsters. You can feel a little tingle, that's magic in action! These brushes are really good at keeping the monsters at bay."

Check: "Next, I'm going to use my sword, also known as a dental probe, to check for any hidden monsters. Not to worry, my sword is very soft and I only use it to gently touch the towers to make sure they are strong."

Finish: "We've done a great job defending your castle! Now, we just need to use some magic water to rinse away any remaining monsters. Then, you can see how shiny and strong your castle looks."

Keeping the history throughout the procedure can make the dental visit more understandable and less intimidating for the child. In addition, it can help the child understand the purpose of each step, which can make him or her feel more comfortable and in control.

End of History

At the end of the procedure, the dentist could cap off the story with a happy ending, saying something like, "We did it. Together, we protected your castle of teeth from the bacteria mons- trues. good job!"

This narrative can help to de-dramatize the dental procedure and make it more understandable and less frightening for the child. By framing the procedure as an exciting adventure, the dentist can help change the child's attitude toward dental visits and make the experience more pleasant and less stressful.

By ending the story in this way, the practitioner validates the child's emotions, reinforces his or her role in the process, and provides an exciting closure that can help reduce any anxiety the child may have. This can make the dental visit a more positive and less frightening experience for the child.

Celebration of success: "We did it. We have successfully protected your castle from the little monsters, the bacteria. Your castle, your teeth, are now stronger and brighter than ever."

Praise to the boy: "And all of this was possible because of your courage and cooperation. You've been an amazing guardian for your castle, and I'm very proud of you. good job!"

Continuous care reminder: "But remember, as the brave guardian of your castle, it's important that you continue to protect it every day. That means brushing your teeth in the morning and at night, and avoiding too many of the sweets that monsters love so much."

Invitation to future adventures: "I hope to see you next time for another exciting adventure to protect your castle. Are you ready for that?"

By concluding the story in this way, the dentist can help the child feel accomplished, validated and excited about future dental visits. This may result in a more confident and less anxious child at future dental visits.

RELIEF OF PAIN AND DISCOMFORT

Pain management is one of the most common uses of hypnosis in dentistry. By helping children focus their attention away from the sensation of pain and toward more pleasant sensations, hypnosis can provide effective pain relief.

Absolutely correct. Hypnosis can be an effective tool for pain management in pediatric dentistry.

Here we explain how it can be applied:

1. Diversion of Attention

The technique of diverting attention is a useful tool in pediatric dentistry used to manage anxiety and fear of pain during dental procedures.

Here is an example of how this technique might be used: The dentist might begin by saying, "I know this may be a problem for you. I may seem a little strange, but I'd like you to do something for me. I'd like you to close your eyes and think of your favorite place in the whole world. It could be a park where you play, a beach where you've been on vacation, or even an imaginary world. I want you to imagine you're there right now."

While the child is visualizing his or her favorite place, the dentist continues, "Now, while you are in that place, I want you to think about how it feels. Can you feel the warmth of the sun on your skin? The smell of the flowers in the air? Can you hear the sounds of the ocean waves or the leaves of the trees rustling in the wind?"

By focusing on these pleasurable sensations, the child can divert his or her attention away from the dental procedure and feel less fear or anxiety.

In addition, the dentist can help the child focus his or her attention on different parts of the body that are not being affected by the dental procedure. For example, the dentist might say, "Now, while you are still at your favorite place, I would like you to concentrate on your hands. Imagine how they feel, how each finger relaxes and how all the tension melts away."

By asking the child to focus on these pleasant images and sensations, the dentist can help take the child's attention away from the dental procedure and reduce the child's perception of pain. This technique, when used correctly, can make the dental experience more comfortable and less stressful for the child.

2. Anesthesia Suggestion

Hypnotic anesthesia" is a technique that can be used by a dentist trained in hypnosis to help minimize the sensation of pain during a dental procedure. Here's how a dentist might do it:

Introduction of the idea

Introducing such a metaphor into the conversation can help children better understand what will happen during the dental procedure and feel more in control.

By presenting the anesthesia as a "super skill" of their own mouth, the dentist can reduce the anxiety and fear associated with the injection or the procedure itself. As the anesthesia begins to work, the child can be encouraged to think that his "superhero" is doing his job, causing the area of his mouth to become "insensi- ble" to protect him from pain.

In addition, this approach can also encourage a positive attitude toward oral health. By encouraging the child to think of his or her mouth as a "superhero," the dentist can reinforce the importance of keeping teeth and gums clean to keep that superhero strong and healthy.

Induction of hypnotic anesthesia

This is an effective way to introduce hypnotic anesthesia. By describing the sensation of anesthesia as a "soft blanket of snow" covering the area, the dentist can help the child associate the numbing sensation with something soft and comfortable rather than something intimidating.

The use of metaphors and visually rich descriptions can help children understand and accept the sensations they are experiencing during a dental procedure. Mentioning "coolness" can also be helpful, as anesthesia is likely to make the mouth feel cool or cold.

Thus, through suggestion and induc- tion, hypnosis can transform the experience of a patient.

dental procedure from something that might be perceived as uncomfortable or frightening, into a more positive and manageable experience. As such, hypnosis can be a valuable tool in pediatric dentistry, helping children manage their fear and anxiety and have more positive dental experiences.

Reinforcement of the idea

This is a wonderful reinforcement strategy. Repeated positive words and affirmations during the dental procedure can help keep the child focused on the "superpower" metaphor, rather than thinking about the procedure itself.

Throughout the procedure, the dentist can continue to encourage the child to pay attention to the sensations of coolness and numbness that his or her "superpower" is creating. This can help minimize any concerns or worries the child may have about the dental procedure.

In addition, this can also make the child feel more in control, as the emphasis is on his or her own "superpower" and how it is helping to protect him or her. This sense of control can be especially helpful in reducing anxiety and encouraging cooperation during dental procedures.

3. Visualization

Visualization is a powerful technique that can be used in hypnosis to help manage pain. Here I show you how a dentist might guide a child in this visualization:

Introduction of the image

In hypnosis applied to pediatric dentistry, an effective technique involves giving the child a clear and manageable image that allows him or her to understand and control the sensations of anesthesia. A frequently used metaphor is that of the "light switch".

A light switch is a familiar object to most children, and its operation is easy to understand. When the dentist presents this image to the child, it provides them with a mental tool that they can use to pro- cess what happens during the dental procedure.

In addition, this switch metaphor promotes a sense of control in the child. By suggesting that the child can "turn off" the sensations in his or her mouth, the child is given the opportunity to feel that he or she has some control during the dental procedure, which may alleviate any anxiety or fear.

Instead of focusing the child's attention on "pain" or "discomfort," the light switch metaphor focuses on "insensitivity." In doing so, it minimizes any possible negative associations the child may have regarding the dental procedure.

As the treatment progresses, the dentist can remind the child of the switch metaphor and reinforce the idea that he or she can "turn off" any discomfort. This helps to consolidate the image in the child's mind and enhance its effectiveness.

Turning off the switch

During the procedure, the dentist can reinforce this image, reminding the child, "Remember, the switch is off. Your mouth still feels comfortable and relaxed, and that feeling will remain as long as the switch is off."

This keeps the child focused on the idea that they are in control of their experience and helps to decrease any anxiety they may have. Even after the procedure, this switch image can be helpful to the child in managing any post-procedural discomfort, allowing him to "flip" the switch again when he feels ready.

Image reinforcement

After the procedure, the dentist may allow the child to "turn the switch back on" when he or she feels ready. This can reinforce the idea that the child has control over his or her own body and sensations, helping him or her to manage any post-procedural discomfort in a way that makes him or her feel empowered and in control.

By implementing these hypnosis techniques in pediatric dentistry, practitioners can create a more positive experience for children, helping to alleviate their fears and anxieties and ensuring that they feel comfortable and confident during their dental visits.

4. Reinforcing Success

Positive reinforcement is a powerful tool to help children build confidence and decrease anxieties about future dental visits.

This could be an example of how the dentist could reinforce the child's success:

Immediate praise

Immediate praise is a powerful form of positive reinforcement. By telling the child that he or she did an excellent job right after the procedure, the dentist is validating the child's efforts and helping the child associate the dental experience with feelings of accomplishment and courage. This type of reinforcement can increase the child's confidence in his or her ability to handle similar situations in the future, which can reduce anxiety at future dental visits. In addition, it can help create a more positive attitude toward dental care in general.

Highlighting the child's ability to manage pain

By highlighting the child's ability to manage pain, the dentist is reinforcing the idea that the child has control over his or her own body and experiences. This can foster a sense of empowerment and self-efficacy, which is the belief in one's ability to handle and overcome challenges.

By acknowledging the child's effort and ability to cope, you can help build the child's confidence in his or her own ability to handle pain and other potentially challenging aspects of dental visits. This may result in a more positive attitude toward dental care and may make future dental visits less anxious for the child.

Create a positive expectation for the future

Creating positive expectations for the future is an effective strategy for reducing anxiety at future dental visits. By reassuring the child that he or she already knows what to do and that the professional will always be there to help, a sense of security and confidence is being built.

This type of commentary not only reinforces the idea that the child is capable of handling dental visits, but also emphasizes that the dentist is a trusted ally in this process. This combination can help decrease anxiety and foster a more positive attitude toward dental care in the future.

An example of how a dentist might use these techniques to reinforce success after a procedure would be:

Immediate praise: "Wow, you did amazingly well, Sofia! You are a real brave girl and you handled this whole procedure like a champ."

Highlight the child's ability to manage pain: "I was really impressed with the way you used your imagination to help you during the procedure. You did a great job of controlling how you felt. You should be very proud of yourself."

Create a positive expectation for the future: "The next time you come, you'll know exactly what to do. And remember, if you ever feel nervous or have any questions, I'm always here to help. Together, we can make your next visit even easier."

These messages will help reinforce the child's self-efficacy, that is, his or her belief in his or her own ability to handle difficult situations, such as dental procedures. This, in turn, can make future dental visits much less stressful for the child.

PROMOTION OF ORAL HYGIENE HABITS HEALTHY

Hypnosis can be a very effective tool to help children adopt good oral hygiene habits. At its core, hypnosis is a communication process that helps people accept new ideas or behaviors. In the case of oral hygiene, it can be used to help children understand the importance of caring for their teeth and adopt healthy practices more consistently.

Positive Suggestions

Positive suggestions are a key part of hypnosis and can be especially effective when used with children. These suggestions might include statements such as "You love the feeling of having clean, fresh teeth" or "Brushing and flossing your teeth makes you feel strong and healthy." When repeated in a state of hypnosis, these suggestions can help children associate caring for their teeth with positive feelings, which can motivate them to maintain good oral hygiene habits.

Visualization

Visualization can also be a very effective technique for encouraging good oral hygiene habits in children. For example, the dentist might guide the child to imagine that he or she is a superhero who fights "sugar bugs" by brushing and flossing. This playful and engaging approach can make dental care more fun and exciting.

Post-Hypnotic Suggestions

After the hypnosis session, the dentist could give post-hypnotic suggestions to reinforce the new habits. They might suggest, for example, that every time the child sees his toothbrush, he will feel a strong motivation to use it.

Routine Reinforcement

Hypnosis can also help reinforce the oral hygiene routine. The dentist may suggest that brushing and flossing are part of the child's daily routine, just like dressing or eating.

It is important to remember that hypnosis must be performed by a trained professional and that each child is unique. Therefore, specific techniques and approaches may vary depending on the individual child's needs. However, with the right approach, hypnosis can be a valuable tool for promoting good oral hygiene habits in children.

HYPNOSIS STEPS TO ENCOURAGE HYGIENE DENTAL

Hypnosis can be an effective tool to help children learn and adopt healthy oral hygiene habits, such as brushing their teeth. Here's how hypnosis could be used to teach children to brush their teeth through visualizations.

Induction and relaxation: The first step is to help the child achieve a state of deep relaxation. Dentists or hypnotherapists can use deep breathing techniques, visualization and relaxation suggestions to achieve this. For example, they might guide the child to imagine that he or she is in a favorite place, such as a park or beach, and to feel the calm and tranquility of that place.

Visualizing plaque: Once you are relaxed, the therapist can guide you to visualize the plaque on your teeth. You might describe it as a "sticky monster" that adheres to your teeth and causes problems if it is not removed.

Visualization of tooth brushing: Next, the dentist can guide the child to visualize the tooth brushing process. They could describe the toothbrush as a "superhero" fighting the "sticky monster," removing plaque from the teeth. They should emphasize the importance of brushing all areas of the mouth, including the back teeth and gums.

Visualizing the end result: Finally, the dental professional can guide the child to visualize how it feels to have a clean, fresh mouth after brushing. They could describe the feeling of freshness and cleanliness, and how this helps keep teeth and gums healthy.

Post-hypnotic suggestions: After the hypnosis session, the dentist might give post-hypnotic suggestions to help the child remember and apply what he or she has learned. For example, they might suggest that each time the child sees his toothbrush, he will remember the visualization and feel motivated to brush correctly.

HANDLING OF SPECIFIC PROBLEMS

Hypnosis can be an effective tool to improve the quality of life of patients.
nd specific problems in the dental office.

Excessive salivation

The hypnosis technique to control excessive salivation is based on the principle of suggestion and visualization. The goal is to help the child feel that he or she has greater control over his or her body and physical responses, which can reduce anxiety and improve cooperation during the dental procedure.

Below is a more detailed approach to how this technique could be applied:

Beginning the session: The hypnosis session begins with the dentist helping the child enter a state of relaxation. This might involve pro- foundational breathing techniques, progressive muscle relaxation, or visualization of a safe and relaxing place.

Introducing the image: Once the child is relaxed, the dentist introduces the image of the faucet. He might say something like: "Imagine that in your mouth there is a small faucet. This faucet controls the amount of saliva you produce, just as a water faucet controls the amount of water that comes out."

Using the image: Next, guide the child through the imagery, saying something like, "Now, visualize how you turn that faucet to turn it off. As you turn it off, the amount of saliva you produce begins to decrease. You can feel your mouth getting drier and drier as you turn the faucet off."

Reinforcing the image: During the dental procedure, you can continue to reinforce this image. You might say, "Remember your faucet. Remember how you can turn it to control the amount of saliva you produce."

Tongue Bites

Hypnosis can be an effective tool to help children avoid biting their tongues during dental procedures. This is a more detailed approach to how this technique could be applied:

Beginning of the session: As with the technique for excessive salivation, the hypnosis session begins with the odontologist helping the child enter a state of relaxation. This might involve deep breathing techniques or visualization.

Image introduction: Image introduction is an essential component of hypnosis. In this case, the image of a fast, agile fish can help the child to visualize his or her tongue as something that can move quickly to avoid danger, in this case, biting during a dental procedure.

The analogy of the fish in a calm pond can help the child relax and feel safe. In addition, by emphasizing that the fish is fast enough to swim away from any threat, the dentist is reinforcing the idea that the fish is fast enough to swim away from any threat.

that the child's tongue can move quickly to avoid being bitten.

Not only can this image help reduce the likelihood of the child biting his or her tongue, but it can also help reduce any anxiety the child may have about the dental procedure. The image of the fish can be a useful distraction, which can help divert the child's attention from any fears or worries he or she may have.

Use of the image: the continued use of the image during the dental procedure helps to reinforce the suggestion and keep the child focused on the image rather than on any possible discomfort or fear.

By guiding the child through the image of the tongue, like a nimble fish, which quickly darts away when the teeth come near, the dentist is helping the child visualize how he or she can control his or her tongue to keep it safe.

Repetition of this image and the association of the tongue with the nimble fish may help increase the effectiveness of the suggestion. Whenever the child feels his teeth approaching his tongue, the image of the fish swimming quickly away may come to his mind, which in turn may cause him to move his tongue to avoid biting it.

Image reinforcement: Image reinforcement during the dental procedure is an essential component of this hypnosis technique. The goal is to keep the image in the child's mind and reinforce the idea that his or her tongue can move quickly to avoid being bitten, just like the fish in your visualization.

Let's go back to the example of the dentist saying, "Remember your fish. Remember how fast and agile it is, and how it always knows how to where to be to be safe. This constant reminder helps keep the child's attention on the fish image, and reinforces the association between the child's tongue and the safe, agile fish.

In addition, these words convey a message of safety and control, two aspects that can help reduce the child's anxiety and fear during the dental procedure.

It is important that these phrases be repeated regularly and consistently throughout the procedure to maximize their effectiveness. Hypnosis requires continuous concentration and maintenance of the image in the child's mind to be most effective.

Fear of Needles

Fear of needles, or trypanophobia, is common in children and adults. Hypnosis can be an effective tool to help alleviate this fear by redefining how the child perceives the needle. Here is a more detailed approach to how this technique might be applied:

Beginning of the session: As in the previous techniques, the hypnosis session begins by helping the child enter a state of relaxation. This may include deep breathing techniques or visualization of a calm place or situation.

Introduction of the image: At this point, the goal is to change the child's perception of the needle, transforming it from something potentially frightening to something much more manageable and less threatening.

By presenting the needle as a small ant, the odontologist is minimizing the perceived threat. Ants are small creatures and, although they can sting, their sting is usually mild and more of a tingle than a sharp, prolonged pain.

By suggesting that the needle is only going to give a "light touch," you are giving the child a manageable expectation of what he or she may feel. Instead of anticipating a great deal of pain, the child may begin to anticipate only a slight tingle, which is much less frightening.

Furthermore, by saying that "ants are small and do no real harm," the dentist is reinforcing the idea that the needle, like the ant, is not going to do significant or lasting damage.

These changes in perception can help decrease the child's anxiety and make him or her feel more comfortable with the procedure.

Use of the image: After introducing the image of the ant, the dentist can continue to reinforce during the procedure. By saying "Remember the ant. Feel how it gives you a little touch, like a slight tingle, but it's nothing to worry about," you are reminding the child of the ant image, and you are reinforcing the idea that the sensation he or she will feel is comparable to the slight sting of an ant, and is nothing to worry about.

Continued use of the image during the procedure helps to keep the image in the child's mind and divert his or her attention from any fears he or she may have about the injection. By keeping the child focused on the image of the ant and its light sting, the dentist can help reduce the child's anxiety and make the procedure a more positive experience.

It is important for the dentist to speak in a calm and reassuring tone throughout the process to keep the child relaxed and receptive to suggestion.

Image reinforcement: hypnosis. The objective is to keep the image in the child's mind and to reinforce the idea that the sensation of the needle is just a small tickle, similar to the touch of an ant.

The dentist may repeat the ant analogy several times during the procedure to keep the child's attention on the image and the associated sensation. For example, you might say, "Remember the ant. Feel how it gives you a little touch, just a slight tickle."

This constant reminder can help distract the child from the procedure itself and focus his or her attention on the image of the ant and the little tickle. This may make the child feel more comfortable and less anxious during the procedure.

It is important to note that hypnosis does not replace the need for local anesthesia or other pain management techniques during dental procedures. However, it can be a valuable tool to help reduce anxiety and improve the child's overall experience.

Restlessness or Inability to Sit Still

Hypnosis can be a very useful tool to help children who have difficulty keeping still during dental procedures. Here is a more detailed approach to how this technique could be applied:

Beginning the session: As always, the hypnosis session begins by helping the child enter a state of relaxation. This may include deep breathing techniques or visualization of a calming place or situation.

Introduction of the image: Once the child is re- lected, the dentist introduces the cloud image. By

For example, you might say, "Imagine that you are lying on a comfortable cloud. In this visualization, the cloud represents a safe and comfortable place. By saying that the child is lying on the cloud, you are suggesting that the child is in a place where he or she can feel totally relaxed.

By saying "this cloud keeps you safe and helps you feel calm and relaxed," the dentist is reinforcing the idea of safety and reassurance. This can help the child feel more secure and reduce any anxiety he or she may have about the dental procedure.

And finally, by suggesting that in the cloud "your body feels so light and comfortable that you don't feel the need to move," the dentist is putting the idea in the child's mind that there is no need to move, which can be especially helpful for children who have difficulty holding still during dental procedures.

These suggestions can help the child reach a state of deep relaxation, where he/she feels safe, comfortable and without the need to move.

Use of imagery: Of course, at this point in the procedure, the dentist is using hypnosis to help the child remain calm and still during the dental procedure. This is done by reinforcing the cloud image that has been previously introduced.

"Feel how the cloud surrounds you, holds you": Here, the dentist is guiding the child to visualize the cloud as an enveloping, supportive force. This image can provide a sense of security, as the cloud is depicted as something that is there to hold the child and keep him or her safe. This can help alleviate any fear or nervousness the child may have about the dental procedure.

"Feel your body become light and relaxed": This suggestion can help the child enter an even deeper state of relaxation. By visualizing their body becoming light, the child can begin to release any tension they may have, which can help reduce any discomfort during the procedure.

"There is no need to move, just enjoy the feeling of being in this comfortable and safe cloud": This is a key statement. By telling the child that he or she does not need to move, the dentist is giving the child permission to completely relax and simply be present in the moment. This can help children who normally have difficulty sitting still feel that they can relax and be still during the procedure.

In summary, the use of cloud imaging during the procedure can help keep the child relaxed, calm and still, which can facilitate a smoother and less stressful dental procedure for all involved.

Image reinforcement: constant image reinforcement during the procedure is essential to keep the child in a relaxed and calm state. This reinforcement can be done in different ways, including:

1. *Repeating the analogy:* The dentist may repeat the cloud analogy several times during the procedure. This may include phrases such as "Remember the cloud. Feel how it holds you and surrounds you" or "Feel how your body becomes light and relaxed in the cloud." This repetition can help keep the child focused on the image of the cloud and the associated feeling of lightness and relaxation.

2. *Comfort reminders:* In addition to repeating the analogy, you can also remind the child of the sensations

of comfort associated with the cloud. This may include phrases such as "Feel how the cloud keeps you comfortable and secure" or "Enjoy the feeling of being in this comfortable cloud."

3. *Reinforcement of stillness:* Finally, you can re-enforce the idea that there is no need to move. This may include phrases such as "There is no need to move. Just enjoy the feeling of being in the cloud."

This technique can help children feel calmer and more relaxed during the dental procedure, reducing the need to move. However, it should always be implemented by a trained professional and with the consent of the child's parents or guardians.

ETHICS AT HYPNODONTICS

The use of hypnosis in dentistry, as in any other medical or therapeutic discipline, must be rooted in sound ethical principles. In this regard, the ethics of hypnodontics adheres to the general principles of medical ethics.

Autonomy and Informed Consent

The principle of autonomy is one of the most important foundations of medical and dental ethics. This principle holds that every individual has the right to make decisions about his or her own body and health care. In hypnodontics, patient autonomy is essential and must be respected at all times.

Informed consent is a critical aspect of patient autonomy. Prior to any procedure

In all dental procedures, including the use of hypnosis, dentists must obtain informed consent from the patient or, in the case of children, from the patient's legal representative. Informed consent is not simply a document that the patient signs; it is a process that involves communication and understanding.

For consent to be informed, the patient should be educated about all relevant aspects of the proposed procedure. In the case of hypnosis, this may include an explanation of what hypnosis is, how it works, how it is used in dentistry, what benefits it may provide, and any potential risks associated with it.

In addition, patients should also be informed about alternatives to hypnosis. For example, if a patient is afraid of dental procedures, he or she should be informed that, in addition to hypnosis, there are other techniques and tools available to manage anxiety, such as conscious sedation, distraction, cognitive-behavioral therapy, among others.

Finally, it is important to note that informed consent is an ongoing process, not a one-time event. Dentists should be prepared to answer any questions that may arise before, during or after the procedure. In addition, patients should always have the right to withdraw their consent at any time, without any repercussions.

Beneficence and Non-Maleficence

The principles of beneficence and nonmaleficence are fundamental in medical and dental ethics and also apply in the field of hypnodontics. Beneficence refers to the obligation to act in the best interest of the patient, while nonmaleficence refers to the obligation to do no harm.

BENEFIT In the context of hypnodontics, benefit involves the use of hypnosis for the benefit of the patient. This may include reducing anxiety and fear, minimizing pain and discomfort, or improving patient cooperation during dental procedures. The goal should always be to improve the patient's experience and provide the best possible dental care. However, the benefits of hypnosis should be evaluated on a case-by-case basis, considering the patient's needs, preferences and circumstances.

NON-MALEEFFICENCE The principle of nonmaleficence means that dentists should do everything possible to avoid causing harm to their patients. In hypnodontics, this means using hypnosis in a safe and appropriate manner. Dentists should be properly trained in hypnosis techniques and should use these techniques with care to avoid any potential harm. For example, hypnosis should not be used to force a patient to undergo a dental procedure against his or her will, as this could cause psychological distress.

In addition, it should be noted that although hypnosis has a very good safety profile and is generally considered to be free of serious side effects, there may be cases in which it is not appropriate. For example, some people may find the experience of hypnosis dis- orienting or unsettling, especially if they have certain mental health disorders. Therefore, dentists should carefully assess the suitability of hypnosis for each patient and should be willing to consider alternatives if necessary.

Justice

Justice, one of the fundamental pillars of medical and dental ethics, holds that patients should be treated equitably and that health care resources should be distributed fairly. When we apply this principle to hypnodontics, we can see that it has a number of profound and significant implications for practice.

One of these implications concerns access to hypodontics. In an ideal world, all patients would have the same level of access to hypodontics, regardless of socioeconomic background, gender, age, religion, ethnicity or other personal characteristics. However, in reality, we sometimes see that hypnodontics can be perceived as a luxury service available only to the most affluent patients. This is a situation that we must strive to change.

Dentists have an important role to play in making hypnodontics more accessible to all patients who could benefit from it. This could involve offering hypnodontics as an option within their routine practice. They could also work to form referral networks, so that patients who need hypnodontic ser- vices can be easily referred to practices that are experts in the field.

Another implication of the principle of justice is that hypnosis should be used equitably. The decision to use hypnosis should not be made on the basis of irrelevant factors, such as the patient's race or gender. Instead, it should be based on the patient's clinical need and suitability for hypnosis. Patients who have the most to gain from hypnosis, such as those with a high level of anxiety, should be considered for hypnosis.

a particularly great need for dental relief or a particularly great need for
pain, they should have the opportunity to benefit from it.

Finally, we must also consider how the benefits and risks of hypnosis are distributed. This is a key aspect of fairness in hypnodontics. The benefits of hypnosis, such as reduced pain and anxiety, should be available to all patients who could benefit from them. Similarly, any risks associated with hypnosis should be clearly communicated to patients so that they can make informed decisions about their care.

Continuous Care

The concept of continuum of care refers to the comprehensive and consistent care that a health care provider provides to a patient over time. In the field of hypnodontics, this means not only employing hypnosis during dental procedures to help manage the patient's pain and anxiety, but also incorporating hypnosis into the patient's overall dental care plan.

The use of hypnosis as a component of con- tinuous care may include:

- Follow-up consultations: After a dental procedure in which hypnosis has been used, the dentist can schedule follow-up appointments to review the patient's progress, address any concerns or problems that have arisen, and adjust the hypnosis approach if necessary.

- Reinforcement of hypnotic suggestions: During follow-up appointments, the dentist can reinforce the hypnotic suggestions given during the dental procedure. This can help maintain the long-term benefits of hypnosis, such as the reduction of pain and anxiety.

- Self-hypnosis training: The dentist can instruct the patient in self-hypnosis techniques that can be used at home to control dental pain or anxiety. This can allow the patient to take an active role in their dental care and provide relief outside of the dental office.

By providing ongoing care, the dentist can not only help improve the patient's dental health outcomes, but also build a relationship of trust and ensure that they feel supported and cared for throughout their dental care process.

Training and Competence

Training and competence are fundamental to the ethical use of hypnosis in dentistry. It is crucial that dentists who use hypnosis in their practice be appropriately educated and trained in hypnotic techniques.

Hypnosis training should include the basic concepts of hypnosis, methods of hypnotic induction, tactics for managing challenges that may arise during hypnosis, and how to incorporate hypnosis into dental practice. This training can be acquired through specialized hypnosis courses, workshops, and training programs. It may also be beneficial to seek guidance from a dentist experienced in hypnosis.

On the other hand, competence in hypnosis is not only achieved through training. It also requires practice and experience. Dentists should rehearse the techniques and use them in clinical settings under the supervision of an experienced mentor or supervisor until they can demonstrate competency. Keeping abreast of the latest advances and research in hypnosis and seeking continuing education to refine and update skills is also part of competency.

It is vital to note that the use of hypnosis in dentistry must follow ethical and professional guidelines, and dentists must respect the limits of their training and competence. In cases where a dentist does not feel prepared to use hypnosis, he or she should refer the patient to a colleague who is qualified to do so.

Honesty and Transparency

Honesty and transparency are essential pillars in the ethics of hypnodontics. It is imperative that dental professionals maintain integrity and clarity in their interactions with patients when it comes to the use of hypnosis.

Essentially, dentists should be candid about their skills and limitations in the use of hypnosis. They should honestly disclose their level of training and competence, the nature of the potential benefits and risks associated with hypnosis, and the role hypnosis plays in the patient's overall treatment plan.

In addition, dentists have a responsibility to be transparent about how they intend to implement hypnosis in the patient's treatment. This translates into explaining clearly and simply what is involved, how it works, what the patient can expect during the session, and how hypnosis is integrated into their treatment plan.

It is equally crucial that dentists be open about the costs that may be associated with the use of hypnosis. They should provide clear cost estimates prior to treatment to avoid any possible misunderstandings or surprises in subsequent bills.

Honesty and transparency not only comply with ethical principles, but also strengthen the relationship of trust with the patient, improving the effectiveness of the hypnosis and the patient's overall satisfaction with his or her care.

Responsibility to Patients

Dentists have a fundamental responsibility to their patients. This responsibility involves not only providing competent and effective dental care, but also ensuring that the treatments and techniques used are the most appropriate for each individual patient.

An important aspect of this responsibility is the careful evaluation of the appropriateness of hypnosis in dental treatment. Although it may be a valuable resource for many patients, it will not be the most appropriate option for everyone. Patients with certain medical or psychological conditions may not be good candidates for hypnosis. For example, people with certain psychiatric conditions, such as schizophrenia, may experience difficulties or complications with hypnosis.

Hypnosis requires a certain amount of concentration and cooperation on the part of the patient, which may be a challenge for some. Therefore, dentists should carefully evaluate the suitability of hypnosis for each patient before proceeding.

If it is determined that hypnosis is not the most appropriate approach, dentists should be prepared to consider and discuss alternatives with your patients. This may include other methods of pain and anxiety management, such as medication, cognitive behavioral therapy or relaxation techniques.

Ultimately, dentists' responsibility to their patients means putting the interests and welfare of the patient first, and this includes making informed and ethical decisions about the use of hypnosis in dental practice.

Informed Consent

Informed consent is an essential component of any medical or dental procedure, including the use of hypnosis. This process involves sharing with the patient all necessary information about hypnosis, including its purpose, the procedures to be followed, the potential benefits, and the associated risks.

Dentists have a responsibility to clearly explain what hypnosis is and how it will be used in the course of their dental treatment. This explanation should address aspects such as the fact that it is not a state of unconsciousness, that the patient will be in control at all times, and that he or she can choose to terminate hypnosis at any time.

Regarding potential benefits, dentists should discuss how hypnosis can help manage pain and anxiety, reduce the need for medication, and improve the patient's overall experience during dental treatment. However, it is also crucial to discuss potential risks, although these are generally low with hypnosis when performed by a trained professional.

Patients should have the opportunity to ask questions and express any concerns they may have. It is important that the dentist listens and answers these questions in an honest and transparent manner. Only after the patient has received all the necessary information and has had the opportunity to consider it should he or she be asked to give consent to proceed with hypnosis.

Proper Use of Hypnosis

Hypnosis, like any therapeutic tool, should be used with integrity, respect, and in the best interest of the patient. The use of hypnosis to manipulate or deceive patients is not only ethically inappropriate, but can also be harmful and counterproductive.

When used appropriately, it can be a valuable tool in dentistry to help patients manage fear, anxiety and pain. But this should always be done with the patient's informed consent and in a framework of respect and transparency.

Dentists should ensure that they are using it in a way that supports and enhances the well-being of the patient. This includes being attentive to the power dynamics in the dentist-patient relationship and ensuring that hypnosis is not used to coerce or pressure patients into any decision or action.

In addition, dentists must be adequately trained in its use. Hypnosis required in a medical or dental setting is a specialized skill that requires training and practice. Dentists should seek quality training and keep up to date on best practices and ethical guidelines for the use of hypnosis, as well as be able to rely on other colleagues (e.g., physicians or psychologists) and refer appropriately if the particular case requires it.

Communication and Follow-up

Communication and follow-up are fundamental aspects of dental care, especially after using techniques such as hypnosis. Once a hypnosis session has been completed, the dentist should take time to talk with the patient about his or her experience.

Asking how the patient feels after hypnosis can provide valuable information about the effectiveness of the technique and can help identify any adjustments that may be needed for future sessions. Some patients may experience feelings of deep relaxation, while others may feel energized and alert.

It is also important to ask about any pre-occupation or side effects the patient may have experienced. Although side effects are rare with hypnosis, they may include such things as dizziness, anxiety or confusion. If the patient has experienced any of these, the dentist should address the problem and consider whether the hypnosis technique needs to be adjusted or an alternative sought.

Finally, the dentist should discuss the next steps in the patient's dental treatment. This may include scheduling future hypnosis sessions, if deemed beneficial, and coordinating any other dental care the patient may need.

In general, communication and follow-up after a hypnosis session are essential to ensure that the patient feels cared for and supported, and to maximize the effectiveness of hypnosis as a dental treatment tool.

APPENDIX

1- APPENDIX ADULTS

HYPNOSIS SCRIPT TO CONTROL ANXIETY IN ADULTS IN THE DENTAL WARD

[Welcome and establishment of trust] [Welcome and establishment of trust] [Welcome and establishment of trust] [Welcome and establishment of trust]

"Hello, welcome to our dental office. I'm glad you decided to come in today. I'm Dr./Dr. [Your Name], and along with my team, we're going to make sure your visit here is as comfortable and smooth as possible. We know that a visit to the dentist can be stressful for some people, but I want you to know that you are in good hands. Before we get started, is there anything you'd like to discuss or any questions you have?"

[Explanation of hypnosis and obtaining consent].

"To help you feel as relaxed as possible, I would like to suggest the possibility of using hypnosis during your visit. Hypnosis is a safe and effective technique that can help you manage any anxiety you may be experiencing.

feeling. It is about entering a state of intense concentration and relaxation, similar to being absorbed in a good book. You will not lose control or be unconscious. You will simply be more relaxed and open to suggestions that can help you feel more comfortable. Do you agree with this?"

[Preparation for hypnotic induction]

"Perfect. Let's get started then. First, I want you to find a comfortable position in the chair. Let me adjust it for your comfort. Close your eyes when you feel ready and begin to concentrate on your breathing. Breathe in deeply, hold for a moment and then exhale slowly."

[Hypnotic induction]

"Imagine that you are standing at the foot of a beautiful, quiet, grassy hill. At the top of the hill, there is a majestic, ancient tree. You begin to walk up the hill, step by step, feeling how with each step you become more and more relaxed and peaceful.

As you climb, you can notice the details of the scene around you: the gentle murmur of the wind in the tree leaves, the warmth of the sun on your skin, the soft song of the birds. You are completely safe and at peace here."

[Deepening of hypnosis].

"When you get to the top of the hill, you sit under the tree. You feel completely calm and relaxed. In this relaxed state, any noise you hear, even the sounds in this office, will only help you relax even more. And if at any time you need to move around to be more coo- mfortable, that's fine too."

THE NEW HYPNODONTICS

[Implementation of hypnotic suggestions].

"Now imagine a warm, soothing light streaming down from the leaves of the tree, filling you with a deep sense of calm. This light has the amazing property of dissolving any tension or discomfort. As you inhale, you feel this light flow through you, filling you with calm. As you ex- halate, any tension or worry dissolves and goes away."

"In this state of deep relaxation, you realize that you are in complete control of your sensations and emotions. You can feel a deep confidence in yourself and in your ability to handle this situation calmly and peacefully."

[Preparation for the dental procedure]

"Keep this sense of calm and control with you as we proceed with your dental treatment. Remember, this is your experience and you are in total control. If at any time during the procedure you feel you need a break, just let me know."

"When I count to three, you will open your eyes, but you will still feel deeply relaxed and at peace. One, two and three... "

[Follow-up].

"How are you feeling, are you ready to begin the dental procedure? Remember that you can return to this state of tranquility at any time by simply walking through this soothing light and your safe place under the tree."

HYPNOSIS SCRIPT FOR ANESTHESIA IN THE MOUTH DURING PAINLESS DENTAL SURGERY

[Home] [Home

"You are already lying comfortably in the dental chair. You can feel how your body is fully supported. Let me invite you to close your eyes and begin to focus on your breathing. Feel how fresh air enters your lungs with each inhalation and how all tensions are released with each exhalation."

[Breathing familiarization].

I invite your attention to focus on the soft, steady rhythm of your breath. Your breath is like an anchor, keeping you centered in this precise moment. Feel the fresh air entering your lungs with each inhalation. Imagine that this air is like a gentle breeze of calm and tranquility filling every corner of your body.

Now, notice how your chest expands slightly as you pull, offering space for that serene air. You can feel how this gentle, rhythmic expansion creates a sense of openness and acceptance in your body.

As you exhale, imagine that you are releasing any tension, any stress that may be in your body. Your exhalation carries with it any restlessness, leaving a trail of deep relaxation in its wake.

You notice how, with each breathing cycle, your body sinks deeper and deeper into a state of serenity. I encourage you to continue breathing in this way, allowing yourself to go deeper and deeper into this state of relaxation with each breath.

Feel how with each inhalation, you are accepting the calm, and with each exhalation, you are letting go of what you no longer need. There is no rush, no pressure. You are just here, breathing, and with each breath you feel more and more relaxed."

[Creation of the secure space]

Now, in this serenity, I would like you to travel with your mind to a special place. A place that for you represents tranquility, security and well-being. It could be a place you already know, a place you have been to at some point in your life and it has made you feel at peace. It could be a quiet beach, a serene forest, a blooming garden, or perhaps a cozy corner in your home.

If you prefer, it can also be a place that exists only in your imagination. This place can have any shape you wish. It can be a castle in the clouds, a bungalow on a desert island, a cabin in a meadow full of flowers or any other place that makes you feel completely safe and protected.

This place is exclusively yours, it is your personal refuge, a space where nothing and no one can disturb you. In this place, you are surrounded by calm and tranquility, and everything in it contributes to your well-being and peace of mind.

Imagine you are there now. Notice the colors, the sounds, the smells of this place. You can feel your body relax even more as you immerse yourself in this tranquil and safe environment. Feel how this place envelops you with its peaceful atmosphere, allowing you to rest and rejuvenate.

This is your place of safety, your personal sanctuary, where you can always return whenever you need a moment of serenity and calm. When you are here, you can feel completely relaxed, protected and safe."

[Deepening of hypnosis].

"In your safe haven, you become aware of a feeling of numbness and deep relaxation that spreads throughout your body. You notice how this sensation moves from the tips of your toes, through your legs, down your torso, your arms, your neck, all the way to your face. This numbness brings you a great sense of calm and well-being."

[Instillation of anesthesia].

Now, I want you to transfer that feeling of deep relaxation and numbness to a specific area of your body: your mouth. Imagine a wave of tranquility that starts flowing from your heart and goes straight to your mouth. It moves gently, enveloping every part of your body where it passes with an incredible feeling of numbness and peace.

The wave of tranquility begins to relax your jaw. Every muscle, every joint of your jaw is softened and released from all tension. You feel your jaw relax completely, allowing you to open and close your mouth easily and effortlessly.

Then, the wave goes to your lips. Imagine that every cell of your lips is bathed in this wave of tranquility, becoming softer and softer and more relaxed. Your lips feel comfortable and relaxed, almost as if they are floating on a cloud of softness.

Finally, the wave of tranquility reaches your tongue. Feel how your tongue rests comfortably in your mouth, how each tongue muscle relaxes and releases. Your tongue feels light and relaxed, and settles into place without any tension or strain.

THE NEW HYPNODONTICS

As this numbing sensation intensifies in your mouth, so does your sense of calm and security. You feel deeply relaxed, safe and at ease. You know that you are in a safe place, that you are taken care of and that everything is going to be okay."

[Loss of sensation]

Now, I want you to imagine a warm, soft light that begins to envelop your whole mouth. This light can be any color you like, whatever color represents the most relaxation and well-being for you. It could be a soft blue, a soothing green, a relaxing gold, choose the color that makes you feel the best.

With each inhalation, this light becomes more intense, shining brighter and brighter. And with each exhalation, the sensation in your mouth begins to fade even more. It is as if the light is absorbing any remaining sensitivity, leaving you with a feeling of total and absolute numbness.

The light continues to shine, enveloping every corner of your mouth. It reaches your gums, your teeth, the inside of your cheeks, your palate, your tongue. Every part of your mouth is now bathed in this soothing, calm light.

You notice how, as the light becomes brighter and brighter, your mouth becomes more and more numb. The sensation in your mouth gradually fades away, until you can no longer feel anything at all. Your mouth is completely relaxed, completely numb.

At this moment, you feel completely calm, completely confident. You know that your mouth is completely prepared for the dental procedure. This feeling of numbness and security accompanies you throughout the entire process, ensuring a comfortable and stress-free experience."

[Conclusion]

"During this entire procedure, you will be in a state of deep relaxation. You will be able to hear my voice and that of my team, but you will feel completely calm and at peace. Your mouth will remain completely numb, allowing the procedure to be performed without pain. When the procedure is over, you will wake up feeling refreshed, rejuvenated and completely at ease."

[End]

HYPNOSIS SCRIPT FOR OPEN MOUTH CONTROL AND TOTAL RELAXATION DURING DENTAL SURGERY

[Preparation and Relaxation]

"You are now in a safe and comfortable place, getting ready for a dental procedure that will be easy and trouble-free. Let's take a journey together, a journey of relaxation and comfort. First, I want you to find a comfortable position in the chair, allowing your body to sink into it. Feel the way the chair supports you and provides a safe and stable place for you."

[Progressive Relaxation] [Progressive Relaxation

"Now, I want you to close your eyes and imagine a warm, comforting light pouring over you. This light begins at the top of your head, relaxing all the muscles in your face and slowly descending to your feet. Feel every part of your body relax with this light. Feel how your mind relaxes, how your body relaxes, how everything in you surrenders to this feeling of calm and peace."

[Hypnotic Induction] [Hypnotic Induction

"This warm, soothing light now focuses on your mouth. You feel how your jaw relaxes, how the muscles in your mouth become soft and flexible. You can feel your mouth open, easily and comfortably. There is no effort, no tension. Your mouth opens naturally and comfortably, preparing for the dental procedure."

[Deepening of Hypnosis].

"Imagine now that this comforting light becomes. a gentle wave flowing from the top of your head to your feet, passing through your mouth. Each time this wave flows, you feel how your mouth opens even more easily, how your body relaxes even more deeply. This wave of relaxation flows again and again, taking you into a deeper and deeper state of relaxation."

[Hypnotic Suggestions]

"Your mouth stays open naturally and comfortably, effortlessly. You feel completely relaxed and at ease. All is well, you are safe. While you are in this state of deep relaxation, any sound or movement around you simply brings you into even deeper relaxation. You feel that you are in complete control. You can keep your mouth open without difficulty, without tension."

[Reinforcement of Hypnotic Suggestion].

"Every time you find yourself in this dental chair, you will remember this feeling of calm and control. You will remember how you can keep your mouth open easily and comfortably, how you can relax deeply. This feeling of control and relaxation will be with you every time you need to open your mouth for a dental procedure."

[Transition to Normal Consciousness]

"Now, as you maintain this sense of calm and control, you begin to return to your normal state of consciousness. You bring with you this feeling of relaxation and the ability to keep your mouth open comfortably. You are ready for the dental procedure, completely relaxed and in control. When you are ready, you can open your eyes, feeling calm, confident and prepared."

This hypnosis script can be used by the odontologist to help patients relax and maintain the mouth open comfortably during dental procedures. Remember that each individual is unique and the script may need to be adapted for each patient.

EXTENDED SELF-HYPNOSIS SCRIPT FOR THE CONTROL OF BRUXISM BEFORE SLEEP

[Preparation and Relaxation]

"It's time to get ready for a deep, restorative sleep. Do everything you need to do before you go to bed. Turn off all unnecessary lights and adjust the temperature to be as comfortable as possible. Now, get into your bed, snuggle into your sheets and settle into a position that makes you feel relaxed and at ease. Let me guide you into a state of deep relaxation, where your mind and body can fully rest."

[Progressive Relaxation] [Progressive Relaxation

"Now close your eyes and take a moment to tune into your breath. Feel the flow of air in and out of your lungs. Imagine that each time you inhale, you are bringing calm and relaxation into your body. And each time you exhale, you are releasing the tension and stress of the day."

"Start with your toes. Feel them loosen and release. This feeling of relaxation slowly moves to your feet, ankles, calves and knees. Feel your thighs relax, the tension fades from your hips and abdomen. The relaxation moves up your back, relieving any tension in your spine. Your chest and shoulders relax, releasing any weight you've been carrying."

[Hypnotic Induction] [Hypnotic Induction]

"Now, focus your attention on the top of your head. Imagine a soft, calm light beginning to descend from there. This light has a magical, relaxing and healing effect. As it moves down toward your face, you feel all your facial muscles relax. Your forehead softens, your eyebrows, your eyelids, your cheeks, everything relaxes."

[Deepening of Hypnosis].

"The light is now directed toward your jaw. You feel it relax completely. Any tension you have been holding in your jaws simply melts away. This powerful beam of light also envelops your neck, your shoulders, your arms, your hands, your whole body, providing a deep sense of relaxation and peace."

[Hypnotic Suggestions]

"Now, in this state of deep serenity, I want you to repeat to yourself, 'Every time I go to sleep, my jaw remains relaxed and calm.' I want you to visualize that your jaw is loose, without any tension. Imagine that you can see and feel how your jaw stays relaxed while you sleep. There is no clenching or grinding of teeth. Instead, you see yourself sleeping serenely, with your jaw loose and relaxed, all night long."

[Reinforcement of Hypnotic Suggestion].

"Every night, when you lie in your bed and close your eyes, this image of yourself sleeping in a relaxed and peaceful way becomes stronger and stronger. This image guides you into a deep, restorative sleep where your jaw remains relaxed, free of any tension or strain."

[Preparation for Sleep]

"With this clear and powerful image of a calm and peaceful night's sleep in your mind, you begin to slip further into sleep. Let us count together, slowly, to five. By the time you reach five, you will be fully immersed in deep, restful sleep."

"One, you are slipping further and further into sleep.... Two, peace and tranquility fills you.... Three, every muscle in your body is completely relaxed.... Four, you feel safe, calm and ready to sleep... Five, you are deeply asleep, your jaw relaxed, your whole body in a state of complete rest."

This script can be recorded for the patient to listen to every night before going to bed. Self-hypnosis requires practice and consistency, and this script should be used over the long term for best results. Each individual is unique, so the script may need to be adapted to the patient's specific needs. Consistency and patience are essential in this process. Over time, you will notice how these hypnotic suggestions help keep your jaw relaxed and improve the quality of your sleep.

2. ANNEX CHILDREN

HYPNOSIS SCRIPT TO CONTROL ANXIETY IN CHILDREN FROM 5 TO 9 YEARS OF AGE IN THE DENTAL WARD

[Welcome and establishment of trust] [Welcome and establishment of trust] [Welcome and establishment of trust] [Welcome and establishment of trust]

"Hello, [child's name]. I'm Dr./Dr. [Your name] and I'm very happy to see you today. You know what? My job is to help make the mouths of children like you very strong and healthy, and while I'm doing this, I want you to feel as comfortable and happy as possible. Would you like to play a special imagina- tion game with me to help you feel more relaxed and fun?"

[Explanation of hypnosis and obtaining consent].

"Well, this special game is called 'relaxation game', where we will close our eyes and imagine ourselves in a very exciting and fun place. During this game, you will always be in control and you can move if you need to adjust your position. Would you like to play this game with me?"

[Preparation for hypnotic induction]

"Now I want you to find the most comfortable position in this special big chair. Now I want you to find the most comfortable position in this special big chair. See how it can be moved up and down? Let me adjust it for you. When you feel comfortable, you can close your eyes and start thinking about your favorite place where you'd like to be playing right now."

[Hypnotic induction]

"Imagine you are in your favorite playground. It could be a colorful park, a magical castle, or even a candy forest. As you think about this place, your muscles relax and you feel very comfortable and safe. This place is all yours and you can do whatever you want here."

[Deepening of hypnosis].

"Now imagine that in your play place there is a special magic item. It could be a magic candy, a magic wand, or even a magic cloak. This object has the ability to make any uncomfortable feeling dis- appear.Can you imagine it?"

[Implementation of hypnotic suggestions].

"Now, every time you feel that something is bothering you or keeping you still, you can imagine using your magic object to make that feeling go away. You can do this as many times as you want, because this object is completely yours and will always be with you when you need it."

[Preparation for the dental procedure]

"With your magic item at your side, you are ready to begin your dental adventure. But remember, if at any time during your adventure you need a break, just let me know."

"When I count to three, you'll be able to open your eyes, but you'll still feel relaxed and in your favorite playground. One, two, and three..."

[Follow-up].

"How are you feeling, are you ready to get started on your dental adventure? Remember you can always use your magic item if something bothers you."

Note: This script is only an example and should be adapted for each individual child. It is important to obtain always obtain informed consent from the child and parent/guardian before using hypnosis and be prepared to adapt or change the approach if the child does not respond as expected.

HYPNOSIS SCRIPT TO CONTROL ANXIETY IN ADOLESCENTS AGED 10 TO 16 YEARS IN THE DENTAL WARD

[Welcome and establishment of trust] [Welcome and establishment of trust] [Welcome and establishment of trust] [Welcome and establishment of trust]

"Hello, [teen's name]. I'm Dr./Dr. [Your name]. How are you today? My goal is to make your experience here as comfortable as possible. Have you ever heard of hypnosis? It's a technique that allows us to relax and focus on positive images that help us to ma- negate any discomfort or anxiety. Is it okay for us to try it?"

[Explanation of hypnosis and obtaining consent].

"Before we start, I want you to know that you are always in control. If something doesn't feel right, you can tell me at any time. The purpose of this is to help you stay calm and relaxed - are you ready to give it a try?"

[Preparation for hypnotic induction]

"All right, now I need you to get comfortable in the chair. You can adjust it to your liking. When you're ready, close your eyes and think of a place where you feel relaxed and happy. It could be a beach, a forest, your room, anywhere you like."

[Hypnotic induction]

"Now, I want you to imagine that you are in that quiet place. Look around you. What do you see? What do you hear? What do you feel? Every detail you imagine will help you relax more and more."

[Deepening of hypnosis].

"While you are in this quiet, safe place, you will notice that your body feels more and more relaxed. Your arms and legs feel heavy and comfortable, and you can feel a sense of calm flowing through your body, from head to toe."

[Implementation of hypnotic suggestions].

"Now that you feel calm and confident, you will find that you can handle any discomfort or challenge. You can even imagine that you have a kind of 'shield' or 'cloak' that protects you from any feelings you don't like."

[Preparation for the dental procedure]

"With this sense of peace of mind and security, you're ready to move forward with dental treatment. If at any time you need to take a break, you just need to let me know."

"When I count to three, you will be able to open your eyes, but you will maintain this sense of calm and security. One, two, and three..."

[Follow-up].

"How do you feel now, are you ready to continue with the procedure? Remember you can always go back to that safe place in your mind if you need to."

Note: This script is only an example and should be tailored to each individual adolescent. It is important to always obtain informed consent from the adolescent and parent/guardian before using hypnosis and be prepared to adapt or change the approach if the adolescent does not respond as expected.

HYPNOSIS SCRIPT FOR OPEN-MOUTH CONTROL AND TOTAL RELAXATION DURING DENTAL SURGERY

(FOR CHILDREN FROM 5 TO 9 YEARS OLD)

[Introduction and Relaxation]

"Are you ready for an exciting trip? We are going to take a trip together to a very special place, where you will feel super relaxed and at ease. But first, I need you to sit comfortably in this big, soft, cloud-like chair. Do you feel it? It's very comfortable, isn't it?"

[Progressive Relaxation] [Progressive Relaxation

"Now, close your eyes and imagine a warm, magical light shining on you. This light starts at the top of your head, travels all the way down your body to your feet. As it travels through your body, every part of you becomes more relaxed, like when you curl up in bed before you go to sleep."

[Hypnotic Induction] [Hypnotic Induction

"This magic light now focuses on your mouth, making it feel soft and relaxed. You can feel your mouth open easily, just like when you yawn before a really good sleep. You don't have to do anything, your mouth opens easily and effortlessly."

[Deepening of Hypnosis].

"Imagine now that this magical light becomes a gentle wave that goes from your head to your feet, passing through your mouth. Each time this wave passes, you feel your mouth open more easily, and your whole body relaxes even more. This wave of relaxation passes over and over again, taking you into a deeper and deeper state of relaxation."

[Hypnotic Suggestions]

"Your mouth stays open easily and effortlessly. You feel very good, very calm. Any noise or movement around you only makes you feel even more relaxed. You have everything under control. You can keep your mouth open easily, effortlessly."

[Reinforcement of Hypnotic Suggestion].

"Every time you sit in this big, comfortable chair again, you will remember this feeling of tranquility and control. You will remember how you can open your mouth easily and without effort, how you can feel so relaxed. And this feeling will be with you whenever you need to open your mouth for us to look at your teeth."

[Transition to Normal Consciousness]

"Now, maintaining this feeling of calm and control, you begin to return to your normal state. You take with you this feeling of relaxation and the ability to keep your mouth open easily. You are ready for us to see your teeth, feeling calm, confident and ready. When you are ready, you can open your eyes, ready for adventure."

This script can be adapted according to the needs and preferences of each child. Imagination and metaphors are very useful at this age to facilitate the process of relaxation and collaboration during the dental procedure.

SELF-HYPNOSIS SCRIPT FOR THE CONTROL OF BRUXISM BEFORE GOING TO SLEEP (FOR CHILDREN FROM 5 TO 9 YEARS OLD)

[Preparation and Relaxation]

"It's time to get ready for a deep and restful sleep. You've finished all the day's games and the lights are off. The temperature is just right, not too cold and not too hot. Now, curl up in your bed, hug your pillow or favorite toy and get into a position that makes you feel comfortable. I'm going to tell you a story that will help you relax and have sweet dreams."

[Progressive Relaxation] [Progressive Relaxation

"Imagine you are in an enchanted forest and you see a her- m butterfly flying around you. This butterfly has a magical power, every time it touches a part of your body, that part relaxes completely. The butterfly begins to fly around your feet, and as if by magic, your feet feel very light and relaxed."

[Hypnotic Induction] [Hypnotic Induction

"The butterfly continues on its magical path and flies around your legs, which relax completely. Your tummy feels light and happy. Your arms feel as soft as clouds. And now, the butterfly touches your face, and all the muscles in your face relax. Your eyes feel heavy and comfortable, your nose and cheeks feel soft, and your mouth and teeth feel calm and relaxed."

[Deepening of Hypnosis].

"The butterfly is now moving toward your jaw. Feel it relax completely. Any tension you may have in your teeth simply melts away. This magic butterfly makes you feel very relaxed and ready to have sweet dreams."

[Hypnotic Suggestions]

"Now, while you are feeling very relaxed, I want you to imagine yourself sleeping peacefully. Your teeth are relaxed, they don't clench or grind, they are just calm and peaceful. You can see and feel how your teeth stay relaxed while you sleep. There is no clenching or grinding. Instead, you see yourself sleeping serenely, with your teeth calm and relaxed, all night long."

[Reinforcement of Hypnotic Suggestion].

"Every night, when you lie in your bed and close your eyes, this image of yourself sleeping in a relaxed and peaceful way becomes stronger and stronger. This image guides you into a deep, restful sleep where your teeth stay relaxed, free of any tension."

[Preparation for Sleep]

"With this clear and powerful image of a calm and peaceful night's sleep in your mind, you begin to slip further into sleep. Let us count together, slowly, to five. By the time you reach five, you will be fully immersed in deep, restful sleep."

"One, you are slipping further and further into sleep.... Two, peace and tranquility fills you.... Three, every muscle in your body is completely relaxed.... Four, you feel safe, calm and ready to sleep... Five, you are deeply asleep, your teeth relaxed, your whole body in a state of complete rest."

This script can be recorded for the child to listen to every night before bedtime. Self-hypnosis requires practice and consistency, and this script should be used over the long term for best results. Each child is unique, so the script may need to be adapted to the specific needs of the child. Consistency and patience are essential in this process. Over time, you will notice how these hypnotic suggestions help keep teeth relaxed and improve sleep quality.

SCRIPT OF ANESTHESIA IN THE MOUTH FOR DENTAL SURGERY IN CHILDREN FROM 5 TO 9 YEARS OLD.

Hello, little adventurer! Did you know that you are a superhero and that this dentist chair is your spaceship? Yes, that's right, you're about to embark on an incredible adventure into the universe of relaxation. And like any superhero, you have special powers. Today I'm going to help you discover your relaxation power. Are you ready? Let's get started!

[Imagine that you are sitting in the pilot's seat of your spaceship, and before you stretches a sky full of stars. Now, I want you to imagine that you are a balloon. What color is your balloon? Is it your favorite color? Does it have a funny design? Every time you take a breath, your balloon inflates a little, and every time you exhale, your balloon deflates. Like a balloon floating in space, light and free. Continue to inflate and deflate your balloon as we travel together on this adventure.

[Creating safe space] Now, on our journey through space, we arrive at a very special planet. This planet is just yours, a wonderful place where you always feel happy and safe. What is your planet like? Is it full of fun toys? Are there many friendly animals running around? In this place, you feel completely relaxed and safe. You find yourself enjoying this wonderful space and feeling more and more at ease.

[It's time to discover your power. I will give you a magic ice cream, but this is no ordinary ice cream. This ice cream has the power to make your mouth feel cool and comfortable, completely relaxed. What flavor is this magic ice cream? Is it chocolate, strawberry or maybe your favorite fruit? Imagine that you are tasting this magical ice cream. With each bite, you can feel how it cools and re-smoothes your lips, your tongue, your gums, every tooth, every corner of your mouth.

of your mouth. Feel the coolness of the ice cream spread throughout your mouth, making every part of your mouth feel more and more relaxed.

[Loss of sensation] Every bite of your macaronic ice cream is not only delicious, but it also makes your mouth feel more and more comfortable and numb. It's a very nice feeling, like when you tuck yourself in your bed and are about to fall asleep, warm and comfortable. Keep enjoying your magic ice cream and notice how, with each bite, the sensation in your mouth fades more and more, until you can no longer feel anything at all.

You're doing great, superhero! Your mouth is now completely relaxed and ready for the adventure of dental work. You know you're brave and strong, and thanks to your superpower of relaxation, you can handle whatever the adventure throws at you. And remember, at all times, your magic ice cream will keep your mouth comfortable and relaxed. Go ahead, superhero, it's time for you to co- mize your mission!"

STORYTELLING

(Create a scenario)

In the heart of a small colorful town, surrounded by high mountains and crossed by a crystal-clear river, lies the Sonrisa Brillante Dental Clinic. This is no ordinary place, it is a magical refuge where baby teeth and permanent teeth live together in peace and harmony. The person in charge of maintaining order in this dental universe is Dr. Cepillo, a dentist known for his gentleness and his magical ability to cure any dental discomfort.

Scene 1

One sunny day, a little boy named Timmy, accompanied by his mother, came into the clinic with a worried look on his face. Timmy had a baby tooth that was really bothering him. His mother had told him about Dr. Brush and how he had the ability to relieve any pain.

Scene 2

Dr. Brush, seeing Timmy's worried face, smiled warmly and knelt down to be at eye level with the child. He told him how the Baby Teeth are like little soldiers who protect the mouth until the Permanent Teeth are ready to take their place. He explained that sometimes these soldiers must retreat so that new, stronger ones can emerge.

Scene 3

Next, Dr. Brush took Timmy to a magical room filled with colored lights and soft sounds. There, he showed him his instruments, which he described as magical tools that he used to talk to the teeth and help them in their transition. He showed her the dental mirror, which he described as a "magic mirror" that allows you to see every corner of your mouth, even the most hidden ones.

Scene 4

After preparing Timmy with a protective vest and sunglasses to protect him from the "magic light rays", Dr. Brush proceeded to examine the stubborn tooth. He did everything gently and carefully, explaining to Timmy what he was doing at each step.

Scene 5

Finally, Dr. Brush succeeded in convincing Timmy's Tooth of Le- che that it was time to retire. With a gentle motion, the tooth was removed, and Timmy barely felt a thing. He looked at the tooth in his hand and smiled, knowing that his Permanent Tooth would soon be ready to take its place.

Conclusion

Timmy left the clinic that day with a new perception of what it meant to go to the dentist. It was no longer a scary place, but a magical place, full of adventures and amazing characters. From that day on, he was always excited to think about his next visit to the Bright Smile Dental Clinic.

(Development of the conflict)

Scene 6

Dr. Brush continued the story, explaining to Timmy that sometimes, little monsters, called bacteria, get into the mouth and can make little holes in the towers of the castle, which are the teeth.

"Look, Timmy," Dr. Brush said, showing an image.

of an enlarged bacterium on its magic screen. "These little monsters are very cunning. They hide in the darkest and most secret places in our castle and start digging tunnels in the towers."

Scene 7

Timmy frowned, worried about the idea of those monsters being in his mouth. But before he could get too scared, Dr. Brush assured him, "But don't worry, Timmy, because that's exactly what we're here for. We have special tools and powers to fight these little monsters and protect our castle."

Scene 8

Dr. Cepillo took a long, thin instrument, which he called "the magic wand of the teeth. He explained that this magic instrument could find the hidden monsters and expel them from the towers.

Scene 9

Timmy watched intently as Dr. Brush carefully filed his teeth with the "magic wand". Although he felt a slight tingling sensation, he knew it was the wand that was driving the monsters out of his mouth. After a few minutes, Dr. Brush announced that they had succeeded in defeating the monsters.

Scene 10

As a reward for his bravery, Timmy received a new toothpaste that had the power to "create a magic shield" on his teeth to protect his castle against future monster attacks. Dr. Toothbrush reminded him to

Timmy who had to use his magic shield twice a day to keep his castle safe.

Conclusion

From then on, Timmy not only lost his fear of going to the dentist, but also became more aware of the importance of maintaining good oral hygiene to protect his "castle". The experience taught him that, although dental visits can be a little scary, they are always meant to keep his smile healthy and protect it from "monsters".

(Involve the child)

Scene 11

Dr. Brush turned to Timmy, his face serious but friendly. "But I need your help, Timmy," he said to him. "To protect your castle and your towers, I need you to be brave. I need you to open your mouth wide, so I can see all the towers in your castle and make sure they are safe.
Can you do that for me?"

Scene 12

Timmy's eyes sparkled. He was excited to be part of the story, to be a character who could help in this important mission. He nodded with determination and sat upright in the chair, opening his mouth wide, ready for Dr. Brush to explore his castle.

Scene 13

Dr. Brush praised Timmy for his bravery and began gently probing with his "magic wand", making sure to

that all the towers were safe from the monsters. As he went along, he kept Timmy informed of everything that was happening, giving him a sense of control and involvement in the process.

Scene 14

Finally, after making sure all the to- rres were safe, Dr. Brush stepped back and smiled at Timmy. "You did very well, Timmy. You are very brave and thanks to your help, your castle is safe."

Conclusion

Timmy felt relieved and proud of himself. Not only had he overcome his fear of the dentist, but he had also played an active role in protecting his own "toothbrush". This story, this scenario that Dr. Brush had created, made the visit to the dentist an exciting adventure instead of something scary. It made Timmy realize that he, too, had a role in caring for his dental health and that being brave and cooperative with the dentist was part of that role.

This story can make the dental visit more understandable and less intimidating for the child by turning the dental procedure into an exciting adventure rather than something frightening.

(*Presentation of the heroes*)

Scene 15

After examining Timmy's castle, Dr. Brush straightened up and turned to introduce his team. "Timmy, I want you to meet my fellow knights. They are also here to help protect your castle."

Next to her was a friendly dental nurse with a bright smile, Nurse Floss, carrying a large roll of dental floss, and a dental assistant with friendly eyes, Assistant Floss, holding a giant toothbrush.

Scene 16

"As your dentist, I am like a knight who is here to protect your castle," Dr. Brush explained, gently tapping his chest with pride. "And Nurse Hilo and Assistant Floss are my faithful companions on this mission. We're going to use our special tools to smoke out those little monsters and make sure your castle stays strong and shiny."

Scene 17

He then showed Timmy the various "magic tools" they were going to use, including the dental mirror, magic wand, toothbrush and dental floss, and explained how each helped protect his castle.

Scene 18

The team worked together to clean and protect Timmy's castle, with Dr. Brush leading the way and Nurse Hilo and Assistant Floss providing support. Everyone moved with care and finesse, making sure Timmy felt comfortable and safe throughout the process.

Conclusion

After that visit, Timmy no longer saw his dentist and his team as intimidating figures, but as heroes, as knights dedicated to protecting his castle. Each visit was an opportunity to meet with these heroes and work together to keep the monsters at bay and his castle safe from the monsters.

secure. This gave Timmy a sense of trust and confidence in his dentist and his team, and made him view his dental visits as an exciting adventure rather than a frightening experience.

(Involve children)

Scene 19

After introducing his fellow heroes and describing the magical tools they were going to use, Dr. Brush turned again to Timmy.

"Now, Timmy, we need your help. You are the king of this castle and we are your faithful knights," he explained, his voice full of seriousness. "To protect your castle, we need you to be brave. We need you to open your mouth wide, so we can see all the towers of your castle and make sure they are safe. Can you do that for us, King Timmy?"

Scene 20

Timmy's eyes grew wide with amazement and excitement at being named king of his own castle. He nodded enthusiastically and prepared to do what was asked of him. He opened his mouth wide, determined to be brave and help his caba- lleros protect his castle.

Conclusion

Involving the child in the story in this way completely transforms the experience of visiting the dentist. What could have been scary and unfamiliar before now becomes an exciting adventure in which the child is not only an observer, but an active participant.

By making the dental procedure a heroic mission and giving the child a crucial role in that mission, the dentist can make the visit much more understandable and less intimidating. The child learns about dental procedures in a playful and creative way, and can associate the dental visit with positive emotions and a sense of accomplishment, rather than fear and anxiety.

This approach can also help foster in the child a positive attitude toward dental health in general and can motivate him to take better care of his teeth at home, knowing that he is playing an important role in protecting his own "castle".

Scene 21

With Timmy ready to assume his role, Dr. Brush gently placed his hand on the little king's shoulder. "So, what do you think, King Timmy?" he asked with a warm smile. "Are you ready to embark on this exciting adventure and become the heroic guardian of your castle?"

Timmy nodded with a bright smile, eyes full of determination and excitement. "I'm ready, Dr. Brush," he said with a determined tone. "Let's go protect my castle."

(Conclusion)

And so began Timmy's exciting adventure. With each visit to the dentist, he became the heroic guardian of his castle, fighting monsters with the help of his faithful knights, Dr. Brush, Nurse Thread and Assistant Floss.

This narrative completely transformed Timmy's experience. Instead of being a terrifying experience, the visit to the dentist became an exciting mission in the that he played a crucial role. By giving Timmy an ac- tive role in the story, Dr. Cepillo was able to alleviate any fear or anxiety Timmy might have, allowing him to feel more in control during the dental procedure.

The visit to the dentist became a story of bravery and adventure, one that Timmy was always excited to participate in. In the process, he learned about the importance of dental health and how his own bravery and actions could help protect his "castle". And although there were still some moments of nervousness and fear, with his team of knights by his side, Timmy always felt ready to face any challenge that came his way.

Thus, the dentist, through storytelling and the child's active participation, transformed the dental visit from a source of fear to an exciting adventure, and helped Timmy understand and appreciate the value of taking care of his dental health.

BIBLIOGRAPHY .

- American Academy of Pediatrics (2019). Guided imagery. At Healthychildren.org: https://www.healthychildren.org/English/healthy-living/emotional-wellness/Building-Resilience/Pages/Guided-Imagery.aspx.
- American Society of Clinical Hypnosis (2021). What is hypnosis? At Asch.net: https://www.asch.net/Public/GeneralInfoonHypnosis/WhatisHypnosis.aspx.
- Barabasz, A. F. and Barabasz, M. (2006). Clinical and forensic applications of hypnosis. Springer Science & Business Media.
- Bernstein, D. A., & Borkovec, T. D. (1973). Progressive relaxation training: A manual for the helping profess- sions. Research Press.
- Best, T. (2010). Guided imagery: A significant mind-body intervention in nursing practice. Journal of Ho- listic Nursing, 28(4), 276-283.

- Brown, R. P., & Gerbarg, P. L. (2005). Sudarshan Kri- ya yogic breathing in the treatment of stress, anxi- ety, and depression: part I-neurophysiologic model. The Journal of Alternative and Complementary Me- dicine, 11(1), 189-201.
- Brown, R. P., & Gerbarg, P. L. (2012). The healing power of the breath: Simple techniques to reduce stress and anxiety, enhance concentration, and balance your emotions. Shambhala Publications.
- Crabtree, A. (1993). From Mesmer to Freud: Magnet- ic Sleep and the Roots of Psychological Healing. Yale University Press.
- Effects of guided imagery on pain and symptoms in persons with cancer pain. Research in Nursing and Health, 35(4), 397-408. Kwekkeboom, K. L., Wanta, B., & Bumpus, M. (2008).
- Eimer, B. N. (2010). Hypnotize yourself out of pain now!: A powerful user-friendly program for any-one searching for immediate pain relief. Llewellyn Worldwide.
- Elkins, G. R. (2010). Expectancy, therapeutic alliance, and hypnotizability: contributions to the hypnoticing process. In The Oxford Handbook of Hypnosis: Theory, Research and Practice (pp. 215-234). Oxford University Press.
- Elkins, G. R., Barabasz, A. F., Council, J. R., & Spiegel, D. (2015). Advancing research and practice: The re- vised APA Division 30 definition of hypnosis. Inter- national Journal of Clinical and Experimental Hyp- nosis, 63(1), 1-9.
- Elkins, G. R., Barabasz, A. F., Council, J. R., & Spiegel, D. (2015). Advancing research and practice: The re- vised APA Division 30 definition of hypnosis. Inter- national Journal of Clinical and Experimental Hyp- nosis, 63(1), 1-9.

- Elkins, G. R., Fisher, W. I., Johnson, A. K., Carpenter, J. S., & Keith, T. Z. (2012). Clinical hypnosis in the treatment of postmenopausal hot flashes: a randomized controlled trial. Menopause, 19(3), 257-266.
- Fung, D., Cohen, M., & Montgomery, G. H. (2013). Hypnosis for symptom management in women with breast cancer: a pilot study. International Journal of Clinical and Experimental Hypnosis, 61(4), 481-494.
- Gauld, A. (1992). A History of Hypnotism. Cambridge University Press.
- Glauser, G. & Madani, M. (2018). Hypnosis in Dentistry and Dental Hygiene: A Review. Dentistry Journal, 6(2), 13.
- Hammond, D. C. (1990). Handbook of hypnotic suggestions and metaphors. W. W. Norton & Company.
- Hammond, D. C. (2000). Hypnotic induction techniques. American Society of Clinical Hypnosis.
- Hammond, D. C. (2010). Handbook of hypnotic suggestions and metaphors. W. W. Norton & Company.
- Heap, M. and Aravind, K. (2002). Hypnosis: Current Clinical, Experimental and Forensic Practices. Taylor & Francis.
- Heap, M. and Aravind, K. (2002). Hypnosis: Current Clinical, Experimental and Forensic Practices. Taylor & Francis. Lynn, S. J. and Green, J. P. (2011). The handbook of clinical hypnosis. American Psychological Association.
- Heap, M. and Aravind, K. (2002). Hypnosis: Current Clinical, Experimental and Forensic Practices. Taylor & Francis. Yapko, M. D. (2012). Trancework: An Introduction to the Practice of Clinical Hypnosis. Routledge.

- Heap, M. and Aravind, K. (2002). Hypnosis: Current Clinical, Experimental and Forensic Practices. Taylor & Francis. Yapko, M. D. (2012). Trancework: An Introduction to the Practice of Clinical Hypnosis. Routledge.
- Heap, M., & Aravind, K. K. (2002). Hartland's Medical and Dental Hypnosis (4th ed.). Churchill Livingstone.
- Heap, M., & Aravind, K. K. (2002). Hartland's Medical and Dental Hypnosis (4th ed.). Churchill Livingstone.
- Heap, M., & Aravind, K. K. (2002). Hartland's Medical and Dental Hypnosis (4th ed.). Churchill Livingstone.
- Heap, M., Brown, R. J., & Oakley, D. A. (2010). Hypnosis and cognitive behavioural psychotherapies: Allies in the treatment of anxiety disorders and response to traumatic stress. Contemporary Hypnosis, 27(4), 216-223.
- Heap, M., Brown, R. J., & Oakley, D. A. (2010). Hypnosis and cognitive behavioural psychotherapies: Allies in the treatment of anxiety disorders and response to traumatic stress. Contemporary Hypnosis, 27(4), 216-223.
- Heap, M., Brown, R. J., & Oakley, D. A. (2010). Hypnosis and cognitive behavioural psychotherapies: Allies in the treatment of anxiety disorders and response to traumatic stress. Contemporary Hypnosis, 27(4), 216-223.
- Hilgard, E. R. (1977). Divided consciousness: Multiple controls in human thought and action. Wiley-Interscience.
- Hilgard, E. R. (1986). Divided consciousness: Multiple controls in human thought and action. Wiley.
- Holmes, D. S., & Burish, T. G. (1981). Imagery techniques in behavior therapy. Journal of Consulting

- Individual difference variables and the effects of progressive muscle relaxation and analgesic imagery interventions on cancer pain. Journal of Pain and Symptom Management, 36(6), 604-615.
- Jacobson, E. (1929). Progressive relaxation. University of Chicago Press.
- Jacobson, E. (1938). Progressive relaxation: A physiological and clinical investigation of muscular states and their significance in psychology and medical practice. University of Chicago Press.
- Jensen, M. P., Barber, J., & Romig, B. A. (2014). Using hypnosis to manage chronic pain. In The Oxford Handbook of Hypnosis: Theory, Research and Practice (pp. 369-385). Oxford University Press.
- Jiang, H., White, M. P., Greicius, M. D., Waelde, L. C., & Spiegel, D. (2017). Brain Activity and Functional Connectivity Associated with Hypnosis. Scientific reports, 7(1), 1-9.
- Journal of the American Dental Association (2008). Hypnosis may reduce pain, anxiety associated with dental procedures. ScienceDaily. Retrieved from www.sciencedaily.com/releases/2008/12/081202102129.htm.
- Kihlstrom, J. F. (2013). Hypnosis. In Oxford Bibliographies in Psychology. Oxford University Press.
- Kilicaslan, A., Cengiz, M., & Gurbuz, T. (2020). Nitrous oxide sedation for dental patients. Journal of Dental Anesthesia and Pain Medicine, 20(1), 1-8.
- Kirsch, I. (1997). Suggestion in the treatment of depression. In I. Kirsch (Ed.), How expectancies shape experience (pp. 129-162). American Psychological Association.
- Kluft, R. P. (2011). Hypnosis and dentistry: A review of applications and implications. American Journal of Clinical Hypnosis, 53(4), 239-247.

- Kohen, D. P. (2008). Hypnotic inductions: Methods, techniques and scripts for building powerful inductions. W. W. Norton & Company.
- Kohen, D. P. (2008). Hypnotic inductions: Methods, techniques and scripts for building powerful inductions. W. W. Norton & Company.
- Krippner, S. (2002). The epistemology and technol- ogies of shamanic states of consciousness. Journal of Consciousness Studies, 9(3), 17-32.
- Kwekkeboom, K. L., Gretarsdottir, E., & Tofthagen, C. (2012). Effects of guided imagery on pain and symptoms in persons with cancer pain. Research in Nursing and Health, 35(4), 397-408.
- Kwekkeboom, K. L., Wanta, B., & Bumpus, M. (2008). Individual difference variables and the effects of progressive muscle relaxation and analgesic imagery interventions on cancer pain. Journal of Pain and Symptom Management, 36(6), 604-615.
- Lynn, S. J. and Green, J. P. (2011). The handbook of clin- ical hypnosis. American Psychological Association.
- Lynn, S. J. and Green, J. P. (2011). The handbook of clin- ical hypnosis. American Psychological Association.
- Heap, M. and Aravind, K. (2002). Hypnosis: Current Clinical, Experimental and Forensic Practices. Taylor & Francis.
- Lynn, S. J. and Green, J. P. (2011). The handbook of clin- ical hypnosis. American Psychological Association. Heap, M. and Aravind, K. (2002). Hypnosis: Current Clinical, Experimental and Forensic Practices. Taylor & Francis.
- Lynn, S. J., & Kirsch, I. (2006). Essentials of clinical hypnosis: An evidence-based approach. American Psychological Association.

- Lynn, S. J., Kirsch, I., Barabasz, A., & Cardeña, E. (2015). Hypnosis as an empirically supported clinical intervention: The state of the evidence and a look to the future. In International Handbook of Clinical Hypnosis (pp. 31-57). Wiley-Blackwell.
- Martin, D. J., Garske, J. P., & Davis, M. K. (2000). Re- lation of the therapeutic alliance with outcome and other variables: A meta-analytic review. Journal of consulting and clinical psychology, 68(3), 438-450.
- McGeown, W. J., Mazzoni, G., Vannucci, M., & Ven- neri, A. (2009). Hypnotic induction decreases ante- rior default mode activity. Consciousness and cogni- tion, 18(4), 848-855.
- Montgomery, G. H., Schnur, J. B., Kravits, K. L., et al. (2013). A randomized clinical trial of a brief hypnosis intervention to control side effects in breast surgery patients. Journal of the National Cancer Institute, 105(17), 1305-1312.
- Moss, A. (1997). Hypnodontics: A Manual for Dentists and Hypnotists. Crown House Publishing.
- Naparstek, B. (2000). Guided imagery for self-heal- ing. Health Journeys.
- Padmanabhan, R., Hildreth, A. J., & Laws, D. (2018). A prospective, randomised, controlled study examining binaural beat audio and pre-operative anxiety in patients undergoing general anaesthesia for day case surgery. Anaesthesia, 73(10), 1248-1256. 11.
- Raichle, M. E., MacLeod, A. M., Snyder, A. Z., Powers, W. J., Gusnard, D. A., & Shulman, G. L. (2001). A de- fault mode of brain function. Proceedings of the Na- tional Academy of Sciences, 98(2), 676-682.
- Raz, A., & Lifshitz, M. (2016). Hypnosis and meditation: Toward an integrative science of conscious plans. Oxford University Press.

- Rossman, M. L. (2002). Guided imagery for self-heal- ing. H J Kramer.
- Sarbin, T.R., & Coe, W.C. (1972). Hypnosis: A Social Psychological Analysis of Influence Communication. Holt, Rinehart & Winston.
- Shenefelt, P. D. (2010). The application of hypnosis in dermatology. Springer Science & Business Media.
- Smith, J. (2011). History of Hypnosis. In Encyclopedia of Human Behavior (Vol. 2, pp. 309-315). Elsevier Inc.
- Smith, J. (2011). History of Hypnosis. In Encyclopedia of Human Behavior (Vol. 2, pp. 309-315). Elsevier Inc.
- Spiegel, D. (1993). Hypnosis. In Annual Review of Psychiatry (pp. 319-329). Annual Reviews.
- Spiegel, D. and Greenleaf, M. (2005). Trance and treat- ment: Clinical uses of hypnosis. American Psychia- tric Publishing.
- Stanciu, C. (2015). Deep breathing exercise. In Stat- Pearls [Internet]. StatPearls Publishing.
- Tinterow, M. M. (1999). Hypnosis: A new tool in obstetric practice. American Journal of Obstetrics and Gynecology, 180(5), 1037-1041.
- Tinterow, M. M. (1999). Hypnosis: A new tool in obstetric practice. American Journal of Obstetrics and Gynecology, 180(5), 1037-1041. 8. Kwekkeboom, K. L., Gretarsdottir, E., & Tofthagen, C. (2012).
- Vincent, J. L., Kahn, I., Snyder, A. Z., Raichle, M. E., & Buckner, R. L. (2008). Evidence for a frontopari- etal control system revealed by intrinsic functional connectivity. Journal of neurophysiology, 100(6), 3328-3342.

- Yapko, M. D. (2003). Trancework: An Introduction to the Practice of Clinical Hypnosis. Routledge.

- Martin, D. J., Garske, J. P., & Davis, M. K. (2000). Re- lation of the therapeutic alliance with outcome and other variables: a meta-analytic review. Journal of consulting and clinical psychology, 68(3), 438-450.

- Yapko, M. D. (2012). Trancework: An introduction to the practice of clinical hypnosis. Routledge.

- Yapko, M. D. (2016). Hypnosis and Treating Dental Anxiety. Dental Economics, 106(6), 50-52.

- Yeates, L. B. (2018). James Braid: Surgeon, Gentleman Scientist, and Hypnotist. Phenomenology and the Cognitive Sciences, 17(1), 63-78.

www.ingramcontent.com/pod-product-compliance
Lightning Source LLC
Chambersburg PA
CBHW071910210526
45479CB00002B/361